THE ANATOMY WORKBOOK

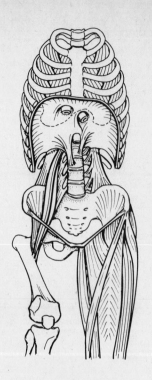

Sandra L. Hagen-Ansert, B.A.
University of California Medical Center
San Diego, California

THE ANATOMY WORKBOOK
A Coloring Book of Human
Regional and Sectional Anatomy

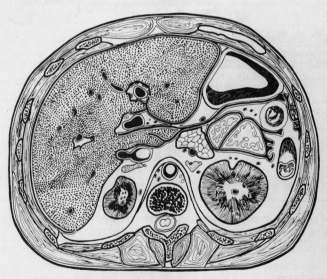

Illustrated by
Jeffrey Allyn Slade

 J. B. Lippincott Company Philadelphia
London · Mexico City · New York · St. Louis · São Paulo · Sydney

Acquisitions Editor: Lisa A. Biello
Sponsoring Editor: Delois Patterson
Manuscript Editor: Lee Henderson
Design Director: Tracy Baldwin
Designer: Earl Gerhart
Production Supervisor: J. Corey Gray
Production Assistant: Kathleen R. Diamond
Compositor: General Graphic Services, Inc.
Printer/Binder: Malloy Lithographing, Inc.

6 5 4 3

Figures 172, 241*A*, 241*B*, and 242 reproduced by permission from
Hagen-Ansert SL: Textbook of Diagnostic Ultrasonography, 2nd ed.
St. Louis, 1983, The C.V. Mosby Co. (241*A* and 241*B* modified from
Townsend CM: Clinical Symposia 32[2]:1, 1980). Figures 243, 251,
and 252 from Bejar R, Coen R: Normal cranial ultrasonography in
neonates. In James HE, Anas NG, Perkin RM (eds): Brain Insults in
Infants and Children: Pathophysiology and Management. Orlando,
Grune & Stratton, 1985, by permission.

**To my daughters,
Rebecca and Alyssa**

Preface

This workbook is designed to provide you, as a student of any imaging modality, with hands-on experience in your effort to learn human anatomy. The anatomical plates are organized according to body systems and organs. Each chapter has anatomical sections that include anterior-posterior views, posterior-anterior views, coronal sections, transverse cross sections, and sagittal sections.

I hope that this workbook will aid you in your understanding of the human body as it is viewed in various projections. If you are a medical, nursing, or health-professional student, you should be able to increase your perception of the human body in a three-dimensional format as you incorporate the anatomical cross-sectional and sagittal illustrations of each organ or structure into your understanding. This conceptualization should help you in understanding and correlating the multiple imaging modalities (x-ray, ultrasound, computed tomography, and magnetic resonance) used today in clinical medicine.

I am indebted to Ellen Mower of the UCSD Office of Learning Resources for providing sagittal illustrations of the human body. I would like to thank Lisa Biello, Delois Patterson, Lee Henderson, and the rest of the staff of J. B. Lippincott Company for their guidance during the publication of this workbook.

Sandra L. Hagen-Ansert, B.A.

Contents

Illustrations

THE ANATOMY WORKBOOK

How to Use This Book

The reader is encouraged to select specific colors for each organ, vascular, or muscular system and to apply those colors systematically throughout the section. Each section and its name should be colored with the same color to allow you to relate the structure and name easily. The specific color assignments are left to your discretion, but it is best to use colored pencils rather than felt-tip markers, which tend to bleed through paper.

Anatomical Terms and Descriptions

Fig. 1 ANTERIOR VIEW OF THE BODY IN THE ANATOMICAL POSITION

Anatomical position (Fig. 1) Standing erect, with the arms by the side and the face and palms directed forward

Median sagittal plane (Fig. 1) A vertical plane passing through the center of the body, dividing it into right and left halves

Paramedian plane (Fig. 1) The plane situated on each side of the median plane

Coronal plane (Fig. 2) An imaginary vertical plane at right angles to the median plane that divides the body into front and back parts (The terms *anterior* and *posterior* relate to this plane.)

Transverse (horizontal) plane (Fig. 1) The plane at right angles to both the median and the coronal planes

Supine Lying face up

Prone Lying face down

Anterior (ventral) (Fig. 2) The front of the body, or in front of another strucutre

Posterior (dorsal) (Fig. 2) The back of the body, or in back of another structure

Proximal (limb reference only) (Fig. 1) Location of a structure closer to the median plane or root of the limb than is another structure

Distal (limb reference only) (Fig. 1) Location of a structure farther from the median plane or root of the limb than is another structure

Superficial/Deep Relative distance of a structure from the surface of the body

Superior (cranial)/Inferior (caudal) (Fig. 2) Levels relatively high or low, with respect to the upper and lower ends of the body

Medial (Fig. 1) Situated close to the median plane

Lateral (Fig. 1) Lying far from the median plane

Internal/External Relative distance of a structure from the center of an organ or cavity

Ipsilateral Located on the same side of the body

Contralateral Located on the opposite side of the body

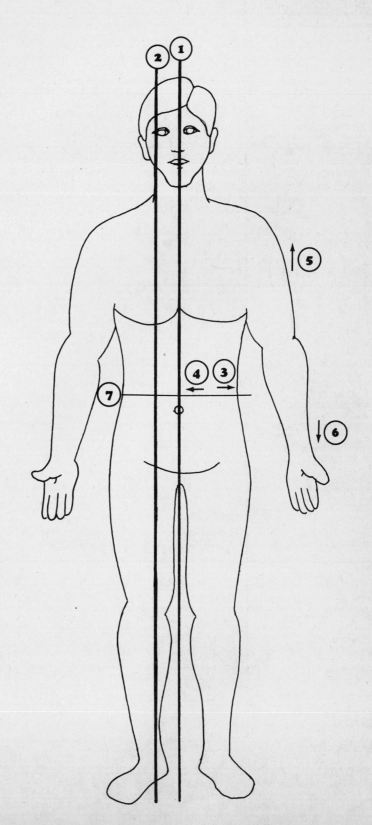

¹Median sagittal plane
²Paramedian plane
³Lateral
⁴Medial
⁵Proximal
⁶Distal
⁷Transverse plane

1

Fig. 2 LATERAL VIEW OF THE BODY

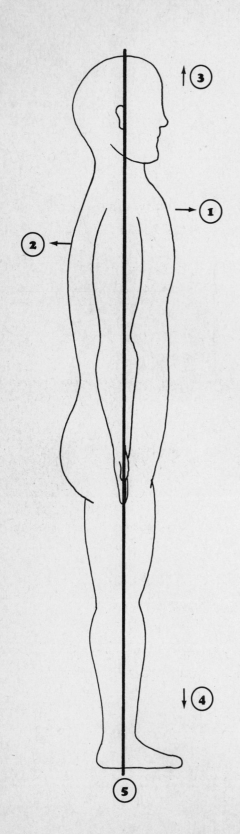

1 Anterior
2 Posterior
3 Superior
4 Inferior
5 Coronal plane

Muscular System
Fig. 3 MUSCLE GROUPS

TYPES OF MUSCLES

There are three types of muscles that can be identified by their structure, function, and location in the body: skeletal, smooth, and cardiac.

Skeletal Muscle (Fig. 3)

The skeletal muscles produce movements of the skeleton and are sometimes called voluntary muscles. Skeletal muscles are made up of striped muscle fibers and have two or more attachments. The ends of the muscles are attached to bones, cartilage, or ligaments by cords of tough fibrous tissue called tendons.

There are four basic forms of dense connective tissue: tendons, which attach muscle to bone; ligaments, which connect the bones that form joints; aponeuroses, which are thin, tendinous sheets attached to flat muscles; and fasciae, the thin sheets of tissue that cover muscles and hold them in place.

The individual fibers of a muscle are arranged either parallel or oblique to the long axis of the muscle. With contraction, the muscle shortens to one half or one third its resting length. Examples of such muscles are the rectus abdominis and the sternocleidomastoid.

Pennate muscles have fibers that run oblique to the line of pull, resembling a feather. A unipennate muscle is one in which the tendon lies along one side of the muscle and the muscle fibers pass oblique to it. A bipennate muscle has a tendon in the center, and the muscle fibers pass to it from two sides. The rectus femoris is a bipennate muscle. A multipennate muscle may have a series of bipennate muscles lying alongside one another (*e.g.*, the deltoid), or it may have the tendon lying within its center and the fibers converging into it from all sides.

Smooth Muscle

Smooth muscle is composed of long, spindle-shaped cells closely arranged in bundles or sheets. Its action—propelling material through vessels or the gastrointestinal tract—is known as peristalsis. In storage organs (bladder and uterus) the fibers are arranged irregularly and interlaced with one another. In such organs, contraction is slower and more sustained to expel contents.

Cardiac Muscle

Cardiac muscle consists of striated fibers that branch and unite with one another. As its name indicates, it is found only in the myocardium of the heart and in the muscle layer of the base of the great blood vessels. Cardiac muscle fibers tend to be arranged in spirals and have the ability to contract spontaneously, and rhythmically. Specialized cardiac muscle fibers form the conducting system of the heart.

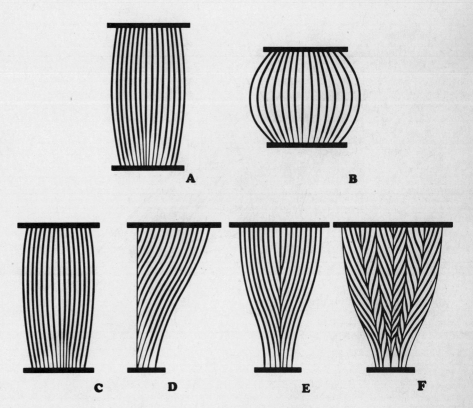

A Resting muscle
B Contracted muscle

Various Forms of the Internal Structure of Skeletal Muscle:
C Parallel
D Unipennate
E Bipennate
F Multipennate

Fig. 4 MUSCULAR SYSTEM OF THE NECK

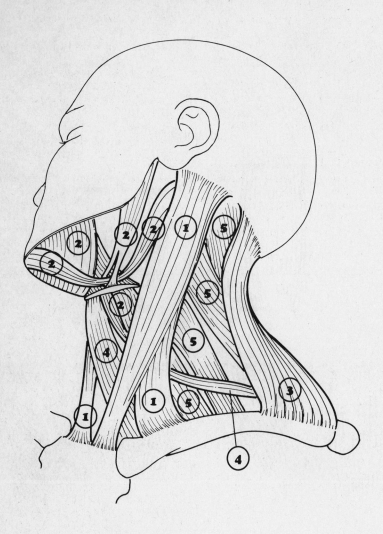

MUSCLES OF THE NECK (Fig. 4)

The neck is a very complex structure, with multiple muscle groups, vascular structures, and fascia interwoven throughout. Only the larger, more superficial muscle groups will be presented here; these will later serve as landmarks for internal structures, such as the thyroid, and vascular strctures found within the neck.

Triangles of the Neck

The neck is divided into anterior and posterior triangles by the sternocleidomastoid muscle; the anterior triangle lies in front of the muscle, and the posterior triangle lies behind.

Anterior Triangle

The anterior triangle contains several important nerves and vessels and is bordered by the mandible above, the sternocleidomastoid muscle laterally, and the median plane of the neck.

Posterior Triangle

The posterior triangle is bounded anteriorly by the posterior border of the sternocleidomastoid, posteriorly by the anterior border of the trapezius, and inferiorly by the middle third of the clavicle. The muscles of this region arise from the skull, the cervical vertebrae, the head of the ribs (scalene), the scapula (omohyoid and levator scapulae), and the cervical and thoracic vertebral spines.

Suprahyoid Muscles

The suprahyoid muscle group consists of the stylohyoid, digastric, mylohyoid, and hyoglossus muscles. The suprahyoid muscles attach the hyoid bone to the floor of the tongue and the mandible. Vessels and nerves to the tongue are found in this region.

Hyoid Bone

The hyoid bone is suspended from the styloid processes of the skull by the stylohyoid ligaments and is stabilized by the suprahyoid and infrahyoid muscle groups.

Infrahyoid Muscles

The infrahyoid muscle group consists of the sternohyoid, omohyoid, thyrohyoid, and sternothyroid muscles. The infrahyoid muscles arise from the sternum, the thyroid cartilage of the larynx, or the scapula and insert on the hyoid bone. Many vessels and nerves traverse this area.

¹Sternocleidomastoid muscles
²Suprahyoid muscles*
³Trapezius muscles
⁴Infrahyoid muscles*
⁵Posterior triangle of the neck

*Anterior triangle of the neck

Fig. 5 POSTERIOR VIEW OF THE TORSO

BACK MUSCLES OF THE TORSO (Fig. 5)

The deep muscles of the back help to stabilize the vertebral column. They also have an influence on the posture and curvature of the spine. The muscles have the ability to extend, flex laterally, and rotate all or part of the vertebral column.

Actions of the Various Muscles

Gemellus superior and inferior: lateral rotator of the thigh at the hip joint

Gluteus maximus: extends and laterally rotates the hip joint; through the iliotibial tract, it helps to maintain the knee joint in extension

Gluteus medius: acts with the gluteus minimus and the tensor fasciae latae to abduct the thigh at the hip joint (important in walking or running)

Gluteus minimus: helps to abduct the thigh at the hip joint; its anterior fibers medially rotate the thigh

Infraspinatus: laterally rotates the arm

Latissimus dorsi: extends, adducts, and medially rotates the arm

Levator scapulae: raises the medial border of the scapula

Obturator internus: lateral rotator of the thigh at the hip joint

Piriformis: lateral rotator of the thigh at the hip joint

Quadratus femoris: lateral rotator of the thigh at the hip joint

Rhomboid: with the rhomboid minor (and major) and the levator scapulae, elevates the medial border of the scapula and pulls it medially

Erector spinae: extend and laterally flex the spine

Serratus posterior inferior: plays a minor role in pulling down the ribs in respiration

Splenius capitis: extends and rotates the head

Supraspinatus: assists the deltoid muscle in abducting the arm at the shoulder joint by fixing the head of the humerus against the glenoid cavity

Teres major: medially rotates and adducts the arm

Trapezius: the upper fibers elevate the scapula, the middle fibers pull the scapula medially, and the lower fibers pull the medial border of the scapula downward.

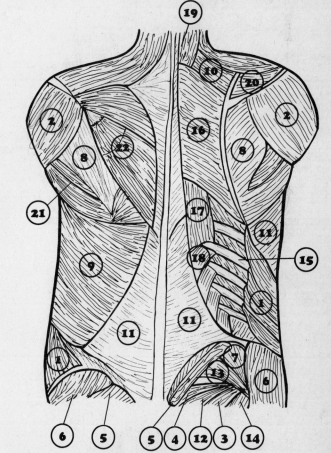

1 External oblique muscle
2 Deltoid muscle
3 Gemellus inferior muscle
4 Gemellus superior muscle
5 Gluteus maximus muscle
6 Gluteus medius muscle
7 Gluteus minimus muscle
8 Infraspinatus muscle
9 Latissimus dorsi muscle
10 Levator scapulae muscle
11 Lumbodorsal fascia
12 Obturator internus muscle
13 Piriformis muscle
14 Quadratus femoris muscle
15 Ribs (7–12)
16 Rhomboid muscle
17 Erector spinae muscle
18 Serratus posterior inferior muscle
19 Splenius capitis muscle
20 Supraspinatus muscle
21 Teres major muscle
22 Trapezius muscle

5

Fig. 6 ANTERIOR VIEW OF THE ABDOMINAL MUSCLES

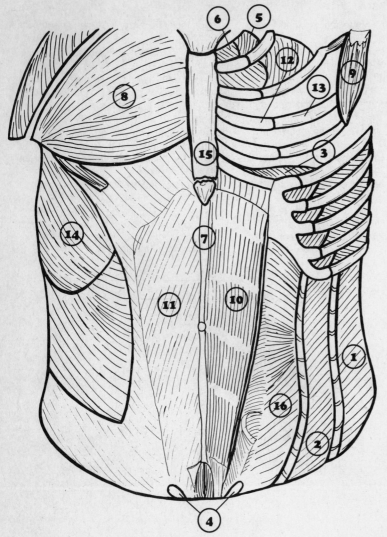

MUSCLES OF THE ANTERIOR AND LATERAL ABDOMINAL WALLS

The muscles of the anterior and lateral abdominal walls include the external oblique, the internal oblique, the transversus, the rectus abdominis, and the pyramidalis muscles (Figs. 6 and 7).

1 External oblique muscle
2 Internal oblique muscle
3 Diaphragm
4 External inguinal ring
5 External intercostal muscle
6 Internal intercostal muscle
7 Linea alba
8 Pectoralis major muscle
9 Pectoralis minor muscle
10 Rectus abdominis muscle
11 Rectus sheath
12 Costal cartilage
13 Rib
14 Serratus anterior muscle
15 Sternum
16 Transversus abdominis muscle

Fig. 7 POSTERIOR VIEW OF THE ABDOMINAL MUSCLES

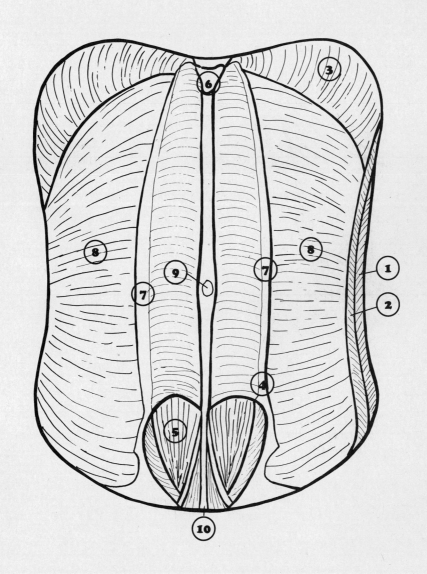

¹External oblique
   muscle
²Internal oblique muscle
³Diaphragm
⁴Linea semicircularis
⁵Rectus abdominis
   muscle

⁶Sternum
⁷Fascia transversalis
⁸Transversus abdominis
   muscle
⁹Umbilicus
¹⁰Umbilical ligaments

Fig. 8 EXTERNAL OBLIQUE MUSCLE OF THE ANTERIOR AND LATERAL ABDOMINAL WALL

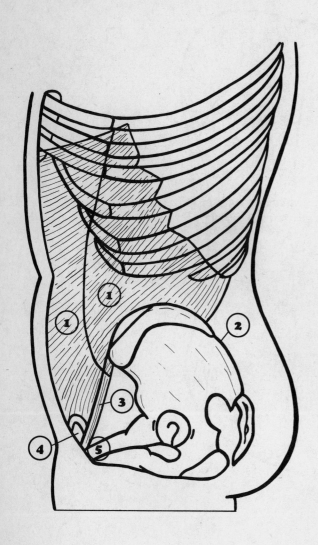

External Oblique

The external oblique muscle arises from the lower eight ribs and fans out to be inserted into the xyphoid process, the linea alba, the pubic crest, the pubic tubercle, and the anterior half of the iliac crest (Fig. 8).

The superficial inguinal ring is a triangular opening in the external oblique aponeurosis and lies superior and medial to the pubic tubercle. (The spermatic cord or the round ligament of the uterus passes through this opening.)

The inguinal ligament is formed between the anterior superior iliac spine and the pubic tubercle, where the lower border of the aponeurosis is folded backward on itself.

The lateral part of the posterior edge of the inguinal ligament gives origin to part of the internal oblique and transversus abdominal muscles.

[1] External oblique muscle
[2] Iliac crest
[3] Inguinal ligament
[4] Superficial inguinal ring
[5] Pubic tubercle

Fig. 9 INTERNAL OBLIQUE MUSCLE OF THE ANTERIOR AND LATERAL ABDOMINAL WALL

Internal Oblique

The internal oblique muscle lies deep to the external oblique; the majority of its fibers are aligned at right angles to the external oblique (Fig. 9). It arises from the lumbar fascia, the anterior two thirds of the iliac crest, and the lateral two thirds fo the inguinal ligament. It inserts into the lower borders of the ribs and their costal cartilages, the xyphoid process, the linea alba, and the pubic symphysis. The internal oblique has a lower free border that arches over the spermatic cord or the round ligament of the uterus and then descends behind it to be attached to the pubic crest and the pectineal line. The lowest tendinous fibers are joined by similar fibers from the transversus abdominis to form the conjoint tendon.

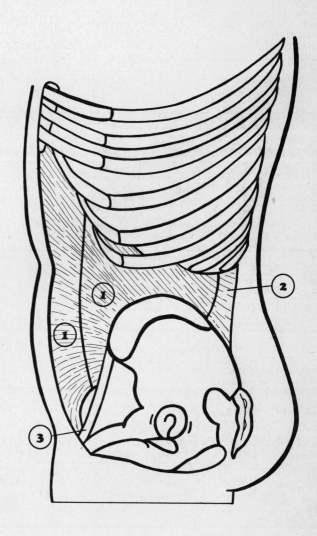

¹Internal oblique muscle
²Lumbar fascia
³Inguinal ligament

Fig. 10 TRANSVERSUS MUSCLE OF THE ANTERIOR AND LATERAL ABDOMINAL WALL

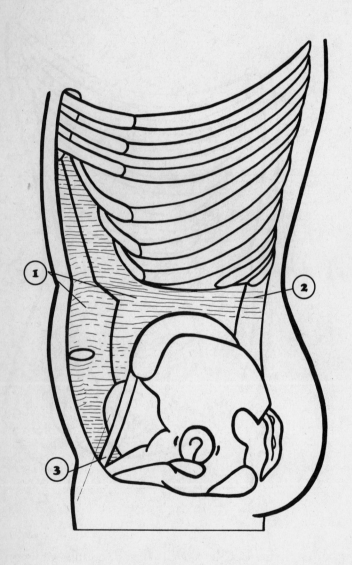

Transversus

The transversus muscle lies deep to the internal oblique, and its fibers run horizontally forward (Fig. 10). It arises from the deep surface of the lower six costal cartilages (interlacing with the diaphragm) the lumbar fascia, the anterior two thirds of the iliac crest, and the lateral third of the inguinal ligament. It inserts into the xyphoid process, the linea alba, and the pubic symphysis.

It should be noted that the posterior border of the external oblique muscle is unattached, while the posterior borders of the internal oblique and transversus muscles are attached to the lumbar vertebrae by the lumbar fascia.

¹Transversus muscle
²Lumbar fascia
³Inguinal ligament

Fig. 11 ANTERIOR VIEW OF THE RECTUS ABDOMINIS MUSCLE AND RECTUS SHEATH

Rectus Abdominis (Fig. 11)

The rectus abdominis muscle arises from the front of the symphysis pubis and from the pubic crest. It inserts into the fifth, sixth, and seventh costal cartilages and the xyphoid process. Upon contraction, its lateral margin forms a palpable curved surface, termed the linea semilunaris, that extends from the ninth costal cartilage to the pubic tubercle. The anterior surface of the rectus muscle is crossed by three tendinous intersections that are firmly attached to the anterior wall of the rectus sheath.

Pyramidalis (Fig. 11)

Although often absent, the pyramidalis muscle arises by its base from the anterior surface of the pubis and inserts into the linea alba. It lies anterior to the lower part of the rectus abdominis muscle.

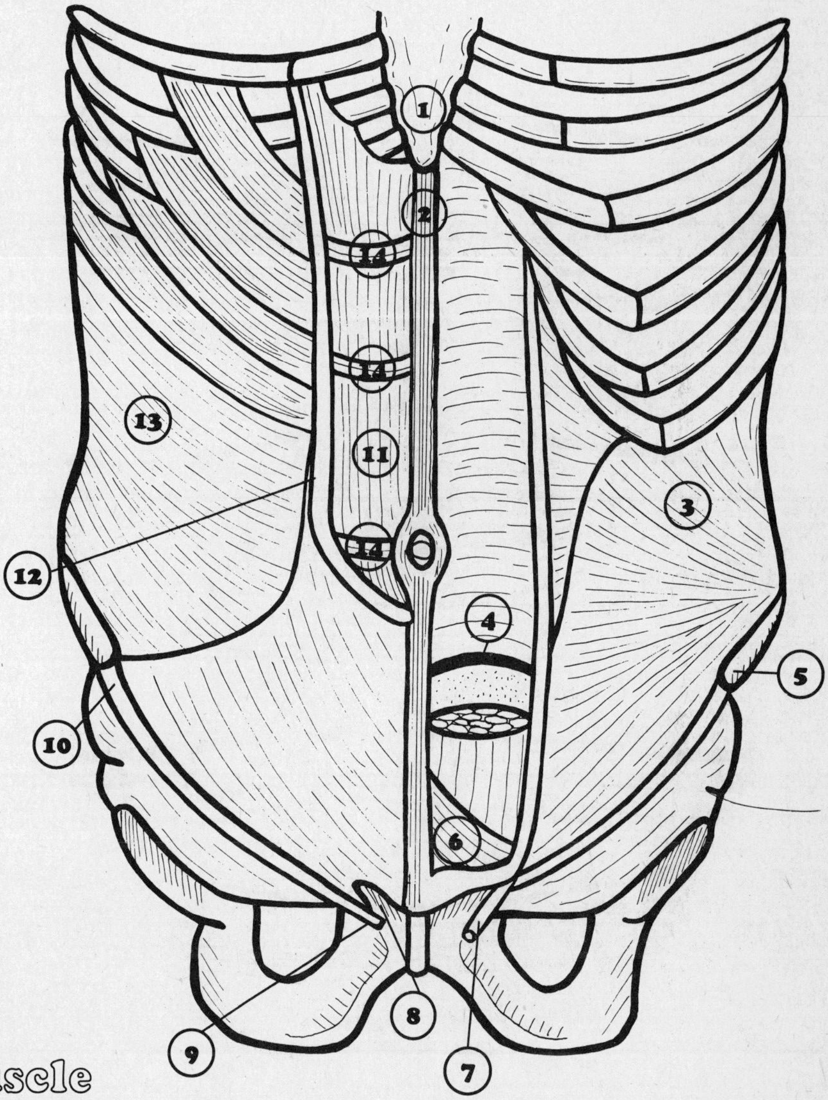

¹Xyphoid process
²Linea alba
³Internal oblique muscle
⁴Arcuate line
⁵Anterior superior iliac
   spine
⁶Pyramidalis muscle
⁷Spermatic cord
⁸Superficial inguinal
   ring
⁹Pubic tubercle
¹⁰Inguinal ligament

¹¹Rectus muscle
¹²Linea semilunaris
¹³External oblique
   muscle
¹⁴Tendinous
   intersections

11

Fig. 12 TRANSVERSE SECTIONS OF THE RECTUS SHEATH AT FOUR LEVELS

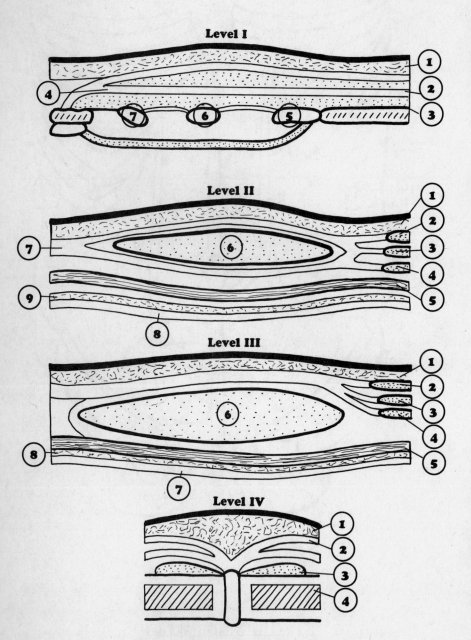

Level I

Level II

Level III

Level IV

Rectus Sheath

The long rectus sheath encloses the rectus abdominis and pyramidalis muscles and contains the anterior rami of the lower six thoracic nerves and the superior and inferior epigastric vessels and lymphatics. It is largely formed by the aponeuroses of the external oblique, internal oblique, and transverse lateral abdominal muscles. It can be divided into four areas:

1. Above the costal margin, the anterior wall is formed by the aponeurosis of the external oblique (Fig. 12, Level I). The posterior wall is formed by the fifth, sixth, and seventh costal cartilages and intercostal spaces.

2. Between the costal margin and the level of the anterior superior iliac spine (Fig. 12, Level II), the aponeurosis of the internal oblique splits to enclose the rectus muscle; the aponeurosis of the internal oblique muscle is directed in front of the muscle, and the aponeurosis of the transversus muscle is directed behind the rectus muscle.

3. Between the level of the anterior superior iliac spine and the pubis (Fig. 12, Level III), the aponeuroses of all three muscles form the anterior wall. The posterior wall is absent, and the rectus muscle lies in contact with the fascia transversalis.

4. In front of the pubis (Fig. 12, Level IV), the origin of the rectus muscle and the pyramidalis (if present) is covered anteriorly by the aponeuroses of the three muscles. The posterior wall is formed by the body of the pubis.

The arcuate line is the point at which the aponeuroses forming the posterior wall pass in front of the rectus at the level of the anterior superior iliac spine. At this point the inferior epigastric vessels enter the rectus sheath to anastomose with the superior epigastric vessels.

The midline linea alba separates the muscles of the rectus sheath. It is formed by the fusion of the aponeuroses of the lateral muscles and extends from the xyphoid process to the pubis.

The anterior wall of the rectus sheath is firmly attached to the rectus abdominis muscle by tendinous intersections, while its posterior wall remains free.

LEVEL I (Above Costal Margin)

1. Superficial fascia
2. Pectoralis major muscle
3. Rectus muscle
4. Aponeurosis of the external oblique muscle
5. External oblique muscle
6. Internal oblique muscle
7. Transversus muscle

LEVEL II (Between the Costal Margin and the Level of the Anterior Superior Iliac Spine)

1. Superficial fascia
2. External oblique muscle
3. Internal oblique muscle
4. Transversus muscle
5. Fascia transversalis
6. Rectus muscle
7. Linea alba
8. Peritoneum
9. Extraperitoneal fat

LEVEL III (Below the Level of the Anterior Superior Iliac Spine and Above the Pelvis)

1. Superficial fascia
2. External oblique muscle
3. Internal oblique muscle
4. Transversus muscle
5. Fascia transversalis
6. Rectus muscle
7. Peritoneum
8. Extraperitoneal fat

LEVEL IV (the Level of the Pubis)

1. Superficial fascia
2. Aponeurosis of the external oblique muscle
3. Rectus muscle
4. Pubis

Fig. 13 INFERIOR VIEW OF THE DIAPHRAGM

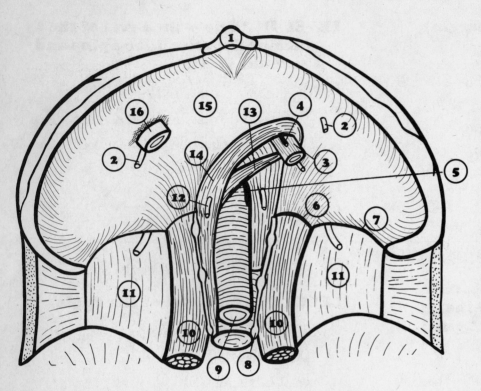

DIAPHRAGM

The diaphragm is a dome-shaped muscular and tendinous septum that separates the thorax from the abdominal cavity. Its muscular part arises from the margins of the thoracic outlet (Fig. 13). The right dome may reach as high as the upper border of the fifth rib, while the left dome reaches the lower border of the fifth rib (Fig. 14).

The right crus arises from the sides of the bodies of the first three lumbar vertebrae; the left crus arises from the sides of the bodies of the first two lumbar vertebrae (Fig. 15).

Lateral to the crura, the diaphragm arises from the medial and lateral arcuate ligaments (Fig. 16). The medial ligament is the thickened upper margin of the fascia covering the anterior surface of the psoas muscle. It extends from the side of the body of the second lumbar vertebrae to the tip of the transverse process of the first lumbar vertebra. The lateral ligament is the thickened upper margin of the fascia covering the anterior surface of the quadratus lumborum muscle. It extends from the tip of the transverse process of the first lumbar vertebra to the lower border of the twelfth rib.

The median arcuate ligament connects the medial borders of the two crura as they cross anterior to the aorta.

The diaphragm inserts into a central tendon (Fig. 17). The superior surface of the tendon is partially fused with the inferior surface of the fibrous pericardium. Fibers of the right crus surround the esophagus to act as a sphincter to prevent regurgitation of the gastric contents into the thoracic part of the esophagus.

[1] Xyphoid process
[2] Right and left phrenic nerves
[3] Esophagus
[4] Vagi
[5] Median arcuate ligament
[6] Medial arcuate ligament
[7] Lateral arcuate ligament
[8] Sympathetic trunk
[9] Aorta
[10] Psoas muscle
[11] Quadratus lumborum muscle
[12] Splanchnic nerves
[13] Left crus
[14] Right crus
[15] Central tendon
[16] Inferior vena cava

Fig. 14 MUSCLES OF THE POSTERIOR THORACIC WALL AND DIAPHRAGM

Openings in the Diaphragm

The aortic opening transmits the aorta, thoracic duct, and azygos vein and lies anterior to the body of the twelfth thoracic vertebra between the crura.

The esophageal opening carries the esophagus, the right and left vagus nerves, the esophageal branches of the left gastric vessels, and the lymphatics from the lower third of the esophagus. It lies at the level of the tenth thoracic vertebra in a muscle sling from the right crus.

The caval opening transmits the inferior vena cava and the terminal branches of the right phrenic nerve and lies at the level of the eighth thoracic vertebra wtihin the central tendon.

In addition to these openings, the splanchnic nerves pierce the crura, the sympathetic trunk passes posterior to the medial arcuate ligament on both sides, and the superior epigastric vessels pass between the sternal and costal origins of the diaphragm on each side.

The left phrenic nerve pierces the diaphragm to supply the peritoneum.

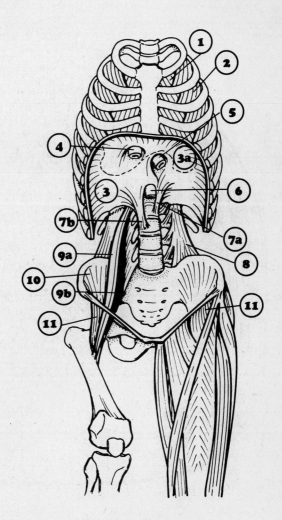

¹Internal intercostal muscle
²External intercostal muscle
³Diaphragm
³ᵃCentral tendon
⁴Inferior vena cava
⁵Esophagus
⁶Aorta
⁷ᵃLeft crus
⁷ᵇRight crus
⁸Quadratus lumborum muscle
⁹ᵃPsoas major muscle
⁹ᵇPsoas minor muscle
¹⁰Iliacus muscle
¹¹Iliopsoas muscle

Fig. 15 CRUS OF THE DIAPHRAGM IN CROSS SECTION

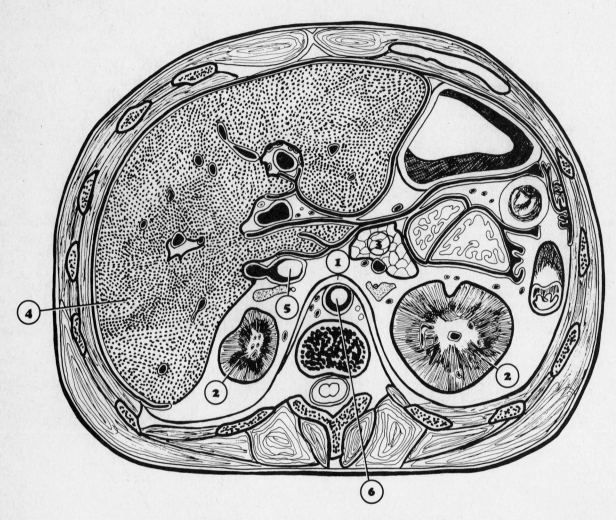

¹Crus
²Kidneys
³Pancreas
⁴Right lobe of the liver
⁵Inferior vena cava
⁶Aorta

Fig. 16 LATERAL VIEW OF THE DIAPHRAGM

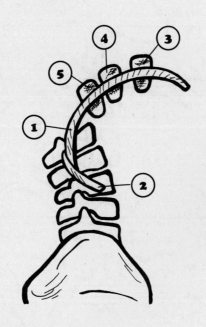

[1] Diaphragm
[2] 12th Rib
[3] Level of the inferior
    vena cava
[4] Level of the esophagus
[5] Level of the aorta

Fig. 17 POSTERIOR VIEW OF THE DIAPHRAGM

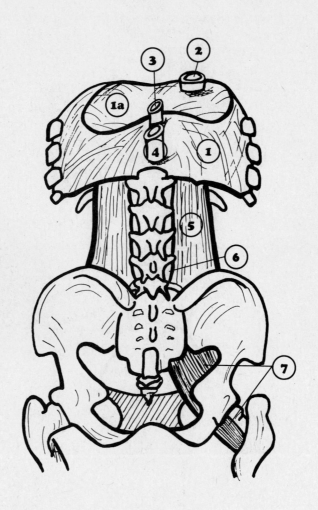

¹Diaphragm
¹ᵃCentral tendon
²Inferior vena cava
³Esophagus
⁴Aorta
⁵Quadratus lumborum muscle
⁶Psoas major muscle
⁷Iliopsoas muscle

Fig. 18 SUPERFICIAL FASCIA OF THE LOWER ANTERIOR ABDOMINAL WALL

SUPERFICIAL FASCIA

The superficial fascia has two layers: the superficial fatty layer (fascia of Camper) and a deep membranous layer (Scarpa's fascia, along the anterior abdominal wall, and Colles fascia, along the perineum) (Fig. 18). The fatty layer may be very thick and is continuous with the rest of the body's superficial fat. The membranous layer fades out over the thoracic wall above and along the midaxillary line laterally. Inferiorly it fuses with the deep fascia just below the inguinal ligament.

Unattached to the pubis in the midline, it forms a tubular sheath for the penis or clitoris. Below, it continues over the perineum and forms a saclike structure for the scrotum or labia majora. It widens in the perineum and attaches to each side of the pubic arch. Posteriorly it fuses with the perineal body and the posterior margin of the perineal membrane.

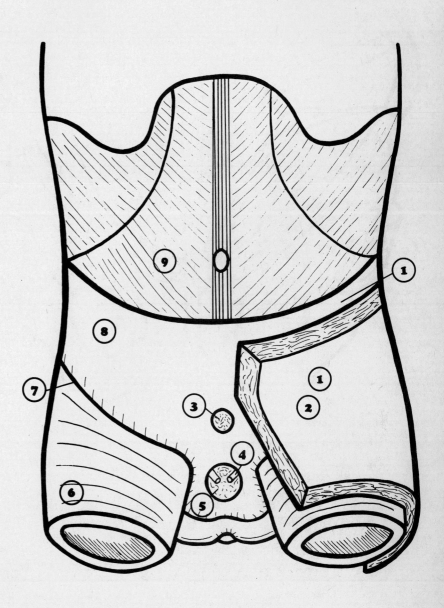

¹Superficial fascia
²Fatty layer (Camper's fascia)
³Position of the penis
⁴Spermatic cord
⁵Position of the scrotum
⁶Fascia lata
⁷Line of fusion
⁸Membranous layer (Scarpa's fascia)
⁹Aponeurosis of the external oblique muscle

Fig. 19 ANTERIOR VIEW OF THE PELVIS

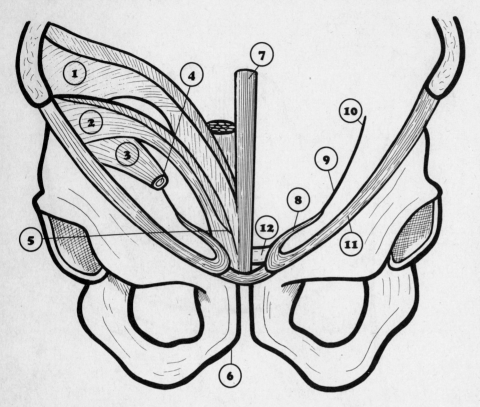

¹Transversus muscle
²Internal oblique muscle
³Cremaster muscle
⁴Spermatic cord
⁵Conjoint tendon
⁶Aponeurosis of the external oblique muscle
⁷Linea alba
⁸Pectineal ligament
⁹Pectineal line
¹⁰Iliopectineal line
¹¹Inguinal ligament
¹²Pubic crest

DIVISIONS AND MUSCLES OF THE PELVIS (Figs. 19 Through 21)

General Features

The pelvis may be divided into two sections: the inferiormost section is the minor or "true" pelvis. The superior section is termed the major or "false" pelvis.

True Pelvis

The true pelvis is bounded posteriorly by the sacrum and coccyx. The anterior and lateral margins are formed by the pubis, the ischium, and a small portion of the ilium. A muscular "sling" composed of the coccygeus and levator ani muscles forms the inferior boundary of the true pelvis and separates it from the perineum.

The true pelvis may further be divided into anterior and posterior compartments. The anterior compartments contain the bladder and reproductive organs (uterus and ovaries or prostate and seminal vesicles). The posterior compartment contains the posterior cul-de-sac, the rectosigmoid muscle, perirectal fat, and the presacral space.

False Pelvis

The false pelvis is defined by the iliac crests, the iliacus muscles, and the upper crest of the sacrum and is actually considered part of the abdominal cavity. The sacral promontory and the iliopectineal line form the boundary between the false pelvis and the true pelvis and delineate the boundary of the abdominal and pelvic cavities.

The uterus lies anterior to the rectum and posterior to the bladder and divides the pelvic peritoneal space into anterior and posterior pouches. The anterior pouch is termed the uterovesical space, and the posterior pouch is the rectouterine space or pouch of Douglas. The latter space is a common location in which fluids such as pus or blood may accumulate.

The fallopian tubes extend laterally from the fundus of the uterus and are enveloped by a fold of peritoneum known as the broad ligament. This ligament arises from the floor of the pelvis and contributes to the division of the peritoneal space into anterior and posterior pouches.

Fig. 20 POSTERIOR WALL OF THE PELVIS

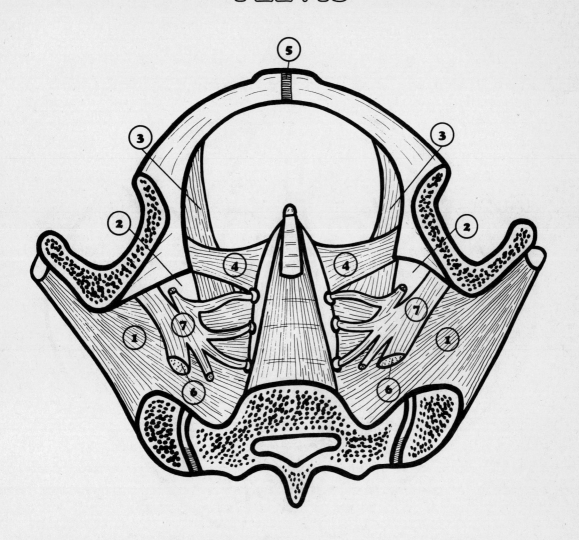

[1]Piriformis muscle
[2]Greater sciatic foramen
[3]Sacrotuberous ligament
[4]Sacrospinous ligament
[5]Pubic symphysis
[6]Lumbosacral trunk
[7]Sciatic nerve

Fig. 21 SUPERIOR VIEW OF THE BONY PELVIS (VIEWED FROM ABOVE)

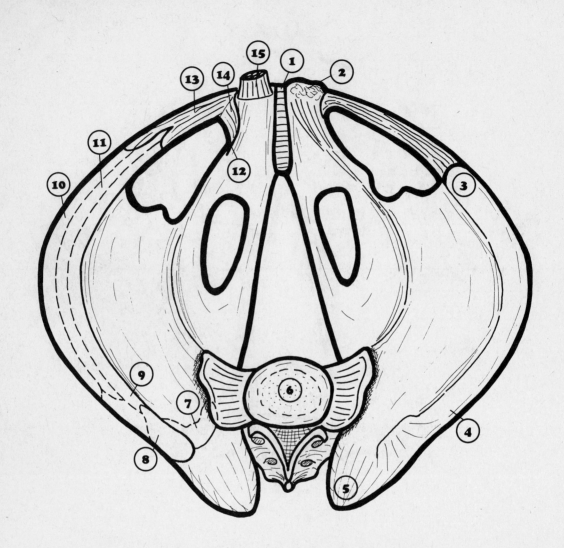

1. Symphysis pubis
2. Pubic tubercle
3. Anterior superior iliac spine
4. Crest of the ilium
5. Posterior superior iliac spine
6. Sacrum
7. Iliolumbar ligament
8. Quadratus lumborum muscle
9. Transversus muscle
10. External oblique muscle
11. Internal oblique muscle
12. Pectineal ligament
13. Inguinal ligament
14. Lacunar ligament
15. Rectus muscle

Fig. 22 INFERIOR WALL OF THE PELVIS

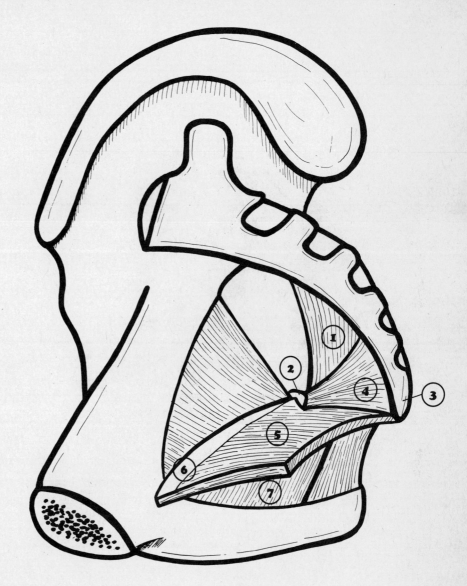

Pelvic Muscles

The posterolateral surfaces of the true pelvis are lined by the obturator internus and pubococcygeus muscles. The obturator internus muscles are symmetrically aligned along the lateral border of the pelvis with a concave medial border (Fig. 22). The pubococcygeus muscles are rounded, concave muscles that lie more posterior than the obturator internus muscles. The psoas and iliopsoas muscles lie along the posterior and lateral margins of the pelvis major. The fan-shaped iliacus muscles line the iliac fossae in the false pelvis. The psoas and iliacus muscles merge in their inferior portions to form the iliopsoas complex. The posterior border of the iliopsoas lies along the iliopectineal line and may be used as a separation landmark of the true pelvis from the false pelvis.

[1]Sacrotuberous ligament
[2]Ischial spine
[3]Coccyx
[4]Coccygeus muscle
[5]Levator ani muscle

[6]Linear thickening of fascia covering the obturator internus muscle
[7]Obturator internus muscle

Fig. 23 INFERIOR VIEW OF THE PELVIS (FEMALE)

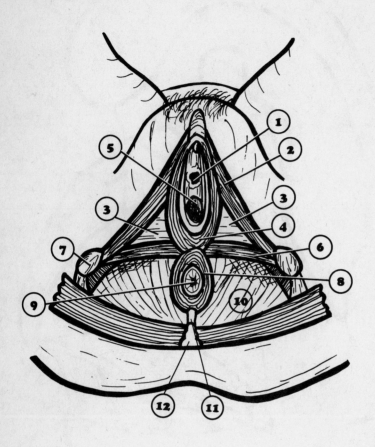

Perineum (Fig. 23)

The true pelvis is subdivided by the pelvic diaphragm into the main pelvic cavity and the perineum. The perineum has these surface relationships: anterior—pubic symphysis; posterior—tip of coccyx; lateral—ischial tuberosities. The region is divided into two triangles by joining the ischial tuberosities by an imaginary line. The posterior triangle is the anal triangle, and the anterior triangle is the urogenital triangle.

The anal triangle has a posterior border of the coccyx, the ischial tuberosities, the sacrotuberous ligament, and the gluteus maximus muscle. The anus lies in the midline, with the ischiorectal fossac on each side.

The urogenital triangle is bounded anteriorly by the pubic arch and laterally by the ischial tuberosities. The superficial fascia is divided into the fatty layer (fascia of Camper) and the membranous layer (Colles' fascia).

[1] Urethra
[2] Ischiocavernosus muscle
[3] Urogenital diaphragm
[4] Bulbospongiosus muscle
[5] Vagina
[6] Transverse perineal muscle
[7] Ischial tuberosity
[8] Sphincter ani externus muscle
[9] Anus
[10] Levator ani muscle
[11] Anococcygeal ligament
[12] Coccyx

Thorax
Fig. 24 EXTERNAL LANDMARKS OF THE THORAX

LANDMARKS OF THE ANTERIOR THORACIC WALL (Fig. 24)

Suprasternal notch: the superior margin of the manubrim sterni. It lies opposite the lower border of the body of the second thoracic vertebra.

Sternal angle (angle of Louis): angle between the manubrium and the body of the sternum. The second costal cartilage joins the lateral margin of the sternum. The angle of Louis lies opposite the intervertebral disc between the fourth and fifth thoracic vertebrae.

Xyphisternal joint: joint between the xyphoid process and the body of the sternum. It lies opposite the body of the ninth thoracic vertebra.

Costal margin: the lower boundary of the thorax, formed by the cartilages of the seventh, eight, ninth, and tenth ribs and the ends of the eleventh and twelfth cartilages.

LINES OF ORIENTATION

Midsternal line (Fig. 24) Lies in the median plane over the sternum

Midclavicular line (Fig. 24) Runs vertically downward from the midpoint of the clavicle

Anterior axillary line (Fig. 25) Runs vertically from the anterior axillary fold

Posterior axillary line (Fig. 25) Runs vertically from the posterior axillary fold

Midaxillary line (Fig. 25) Runs vertically from a point midway between the anterior and posterior axillary folds

Scapular line (Fig. 26) Runs vertically on the posterior wall of the thorax, passing through the inferior angle of the scapula (with the arms down)

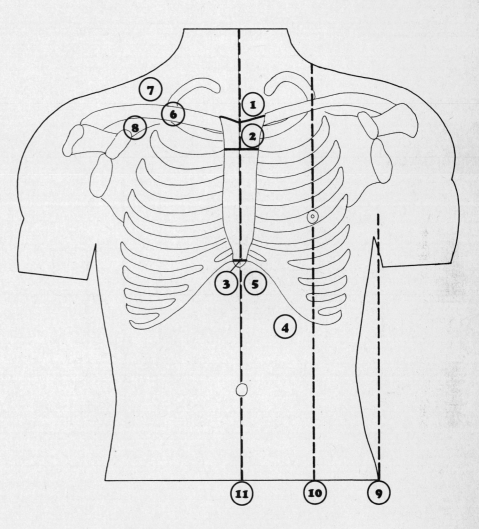

[1] Suprasternal notch
[2] Sternal angle
[3] Xyphisternal joint
[4] Costal margin
[5] Subcostal margin
[6] Clavicle
[7] Supraclavicular fossa
[8] Infraclavicular fossa
[9] Anterior axillary line
[10] Midclavicular line
[11] Midsternal line

Fig. 25 REFERENCE LINES ON THE LATERAL CHEST WALL

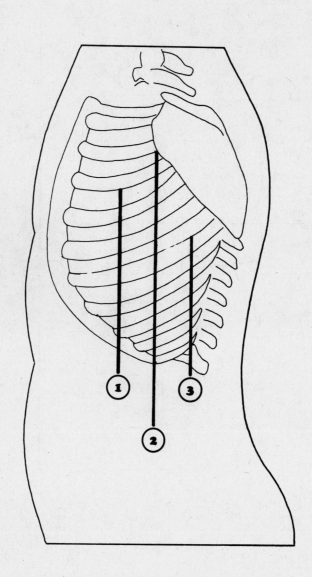

[1]Anterior axillary line
[2]Midaxillary line
[3]Posterior axillary line

Fig. 26 REFERENCE LINES ON THE POSTERIOR CHEST WALL

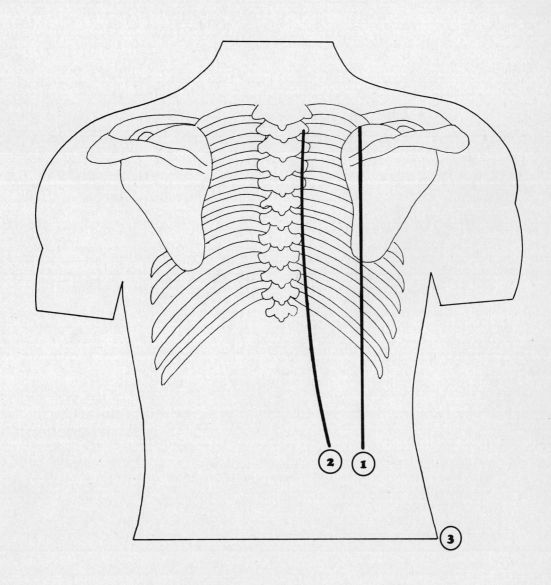

[1]Scapular line
[2]Paravertebral line
[3]Iliac crest

Fig. 27 ANTERIOR VIEW OF THE THORAX

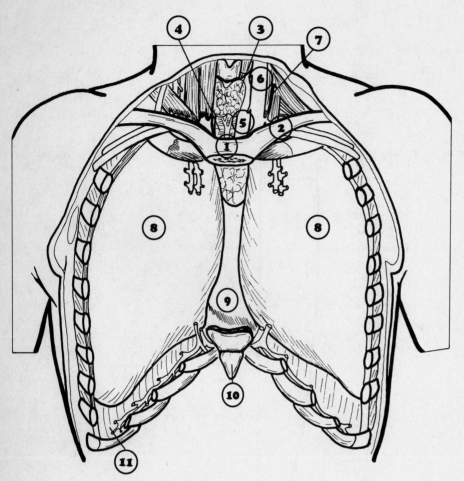

THORACIC CAVITY

The thoracic cavity lies within the thorax and is separated from the abdominal cavity by the diaphragm. For purposes of study, it may be divided into two parts. The mediastinum is the medial portion, while the pleurae and lungs are its lateral components (Fig. 27).

The sternum consists of three sections: the manubrium, the body, and the xyphoid process. The junction between the manubrium and the body of the sternum is known as the angle of Louis and is a useful landmark in locating the cartilages of the second rib or the position of the superior medistinum.

Mediastinum

The mediastinum extends superiorly to the thoracic inlet and to the root of the neck and inferiorly to the diaphragm. Anteriorly it extends to the sternum, posteriorly to the thoracic vertebrae. Within the mediastinum are these structures:

Thymus (remains)
Heart and great vessels
Trachea and esophagus
Thoracic duct and lymph nodes
Vagus and phrenic nerves
Sympathetic trunks

[1] Manubrium of the sternum
[2] Right clavicle
[3] Thyroid gland
[4] Trachea
[5] Left common carotid artery
[6] Left internal jugular vein
[7] Left phrenic nerve
[8] Superior and inferior lobes of the lung
[9] Pericardium
[10] Xyphoid process
[11] Diaphragm

Fig. 28 ANTERIOR VIEW OF THE THORAX WITH THE LUNGS REMOVED

Pleurae

Each pleural sac has two parts: a parietal layer and a visceral layer. The parietal layer lines the thoracic wall, covering the diaphragm and the lateral aspect of the mediastinum, and extends to the root of the neck to line the undersurface of the suprapleural membrane at the thoracic inlet (Figs. 28 through 30). The visceral layer covers the outer surfaces of the lungs and extends into the interlobar fissures.

The two layers become continuous with each other by a "cuff" of pleura that surrounds the structures at the lung root (near the bronchi).

A pleural cavity separates the parietal and visceral layers of pleura with a small amount of pleural fluid. This fluid covers the pleura with a thin coating and permits the layers to move on each other with minimal friction. The costophrenic sinus is the pleural reflection between the costal and diaphragmatic portions of the parietal pleura. This space lies lower than the edge of the lung and is generally unoccupied by lung. Thus, when pleural fluid accumulates, its most common location is in the costophrenic sinus.

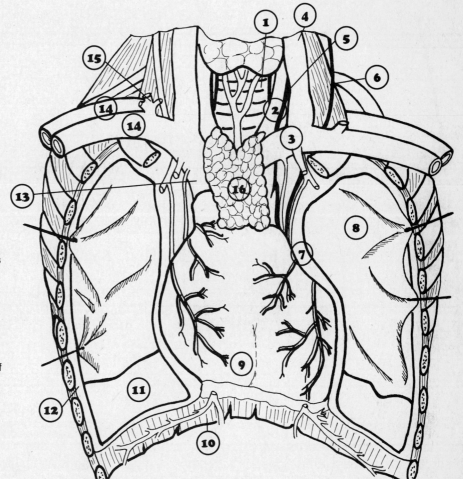

¹Trachea
²Left common carotid artery
³Left brachiocephalic (innominate) vein
⁴Left internal jugular vein
⁵Left vagus nerve
⁶Left phrenic nerve
⁷Mediastinal pleura
⁸Left lung

⁹Pericardium
¹⁰Diaphragm
¹¹Diaphragmatic pleural space
¹²Costal pleural space
¹³Superior vena cava
¹⁴Right subclavian artery and vein
¹⁵Right external jugular vein
¹⁶Thymus gland

Fig. 29 RIGHT LATERAL VIEW OF THE THORAX

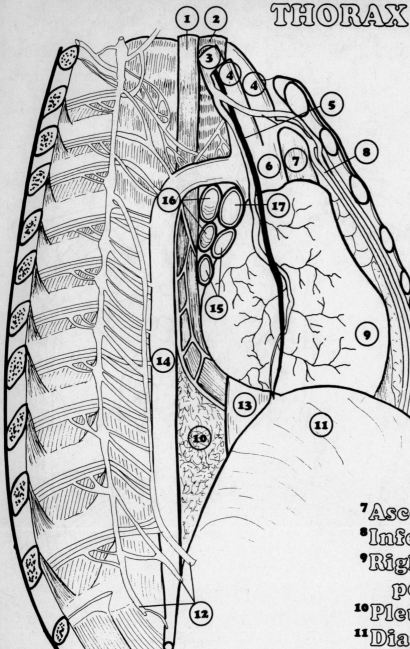

1 Esophagus
2 Trachea
3 Brachiocephalic artery
4 Right and left brachiocephalic veins
5 Right phrenic nerve and inferior thoracic artery
6 Superior vena cava
7 Ascending aorta
8 Inferior thoracic vein
9 Right surface of the pericardium
10 Pleura of the left side
11 Diaphragm pulled inferiorly
12 Greater, lesser, and lowest splanchnic nerves
13 Inferior vena cava
14 Azygos vein
15 Right pulmonary veins
16 Right bronchus
17 Right pulmonary artery

Fig. 30 LEFT LATERAL VIEW OF THE THORAX

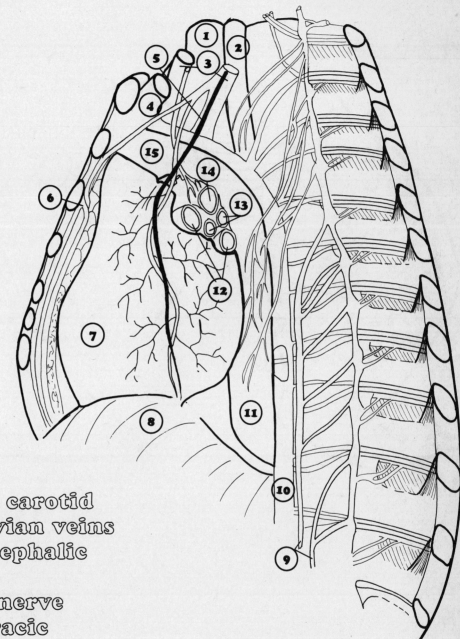

[1] Trachea
[2] Esophagus
[3] Left common carotid and subclavian veins
[4] Left brachiocephalic vein
[5] Left phrenic nerve
[6] Internal thoracic vessels
[7] Left surface of the pericardium
[8] Diaphragm
[9] Greater and lesser splanchnic nerves
[10] Hemiazygos vein
[11] Descending aorta
[12] Left pulmonary vein
[13] Left bronchus (divided)
[14] Left pulmonary artery
[15] Aortic arch

Fig. 31 ANTERIOR VIEW OF THE TRACHEA AND LUNGS

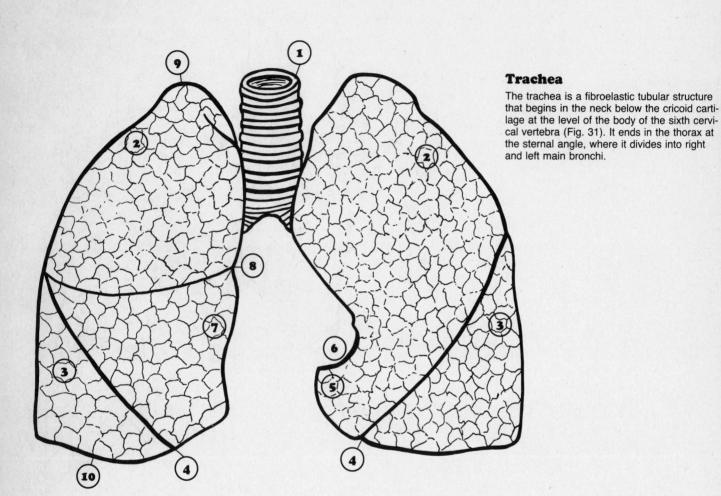

Trachea

The trachea is a fibroelastic tubular structure that begins in the neck below the cricoid cartilage at the level of the body of the sixth cervical vertebra (Fig. 31). It ends in the thorax at the sternal angle, where it divides into right and left main bronchi.

¹Trachea
²Superior lobe
³Inferior lobe
⁴Oblique fissure
⁵Lingula

⁶Cardiac notch
⁷Middle lobe
⁸Horizontal fissure
⁹Apex of the lung
¹⁰Base of the lung

Fig. 32 ANTERIOR VIEW OF THE BRONCHI AND VESSELS OF THE RIGHT LUNG

Main Bronchi

The right main bronchus (Fig. 32) is wider, shorter, and more vertical than the left. The left main bronchus (Fig. 33) passes to the left and downward below the aortic arch anterior to the esophagus before entering the lung.

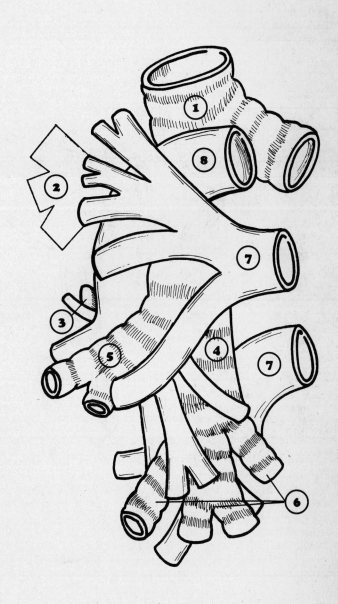

¹Principal bronchus
²Upper-lobe bronchus
³Superior bronchus
⁴Inferior-lobe bronchus
⁵Middle-lobe bronchus
⁶Basal bronchi
⁷Superior pulmonary vein
⁸Right pulmonary artery

Fig. 33 ANTERIOR VIEW OF THE BRONCHI AND VESSELS OF THE LEFT LUNG

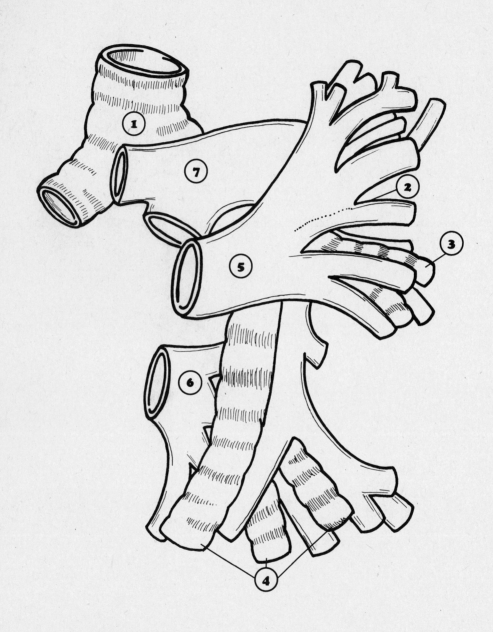

¹Principal bronchus
²Upper-lobe bronchus
³Lower (lingular) division
⁴Lower-lobe bronchi

⁵Superior pulmonary vein
⁶Inferior pulmonary vein
⁷Left pulmonary arteries

Fig. 34 RIGHT LUNG

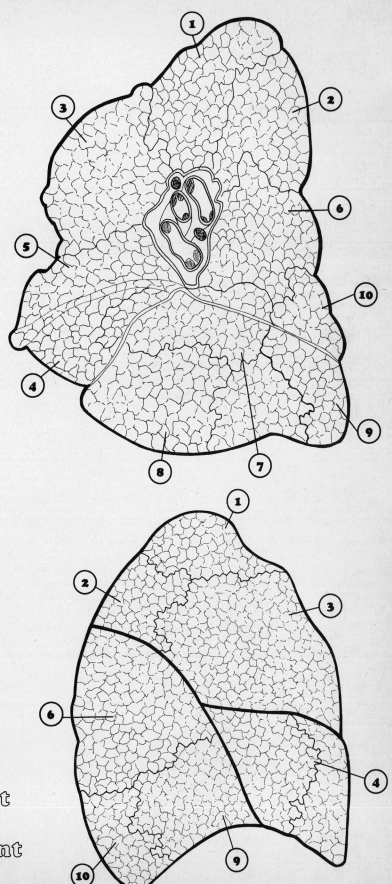

Lungs

Each lung is covered by visceral pleura, suspended in its own pleural cavity, and attached to the mediastinum by its root. Each has a blunt apex, a concave base, a convex costal surface, and a concave mediastinal surface.

The larger, right lung (Fig. 34) is divided by the oblique and horizontal fissures into three lobes: upper, middle, and lower. The left lung (Fig. 35) is divided by the oblique fissure into two lobes: upper and lower.

The lobes are further subdivided into several bronchopulmonary segments that receive a segmental bronchus, an artery, and a vein. These pyramidal segments project their apices toward the root of the lung and their bases toward the lung surface.

The root of the lung is composed of bronchi, pulmonary artery and veins, lymph vessels, bronchial vessels, and nerves. Pleural sheath surrounds it to join the mediastinal parietal pleura to the visceral pleura that covers the lungs.

Superior lobe

^{1}Apical segment
^{2}Posterior segment
^{3}Anterior segment

Middle lobe

^{4}Lateral segment
^{5}Medial segment

Inferior lobe

^{6}Apical segment
^{7}Basal medial segment
^{8}Basal anterior segment
^{9}Basal lateral segment
^{10}Basal posterior segment

35

Fig. 35 LEFT LUNG

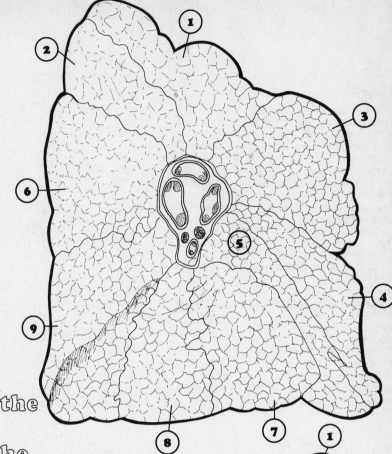

Superior lobe

[1]Apical segment
[2]Posterior segment
[3]Anterior segment
[4]Superior segment of the lingula
[5]Inferior segment of the lingula

Inferior lobe

[6]Apical lower segment
[7]Basal anterior segment
[8]Basal lateral segment
[9]Basal posterior segment

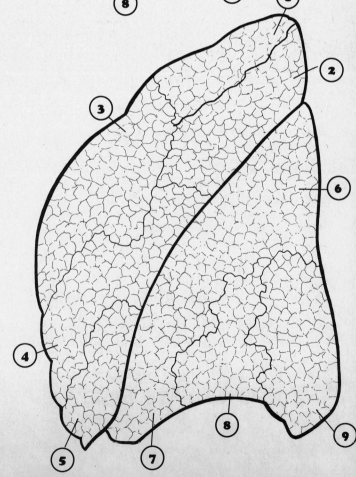

Fig. 36A HEART

HEART AND GREAT VESSELS

The heart lies in the middle mediastinum within the pericardial sac. In addition to its apex, it has three surfaces: sternocostal, diaphragmatic, and base (Fig. 36A).

The sternocostal (anterior) surface is formed by the right atrium (right border) and right ventricle. The vertical atrioventricular groove separates these two structures. The left border is formed by the left ventricle and auricle (the left atrial appendage). The anterior interventricular groove separates the right and left ventricles (Fig. 36B).

The diaphragmatic (inferior) surface (Fig. 37) is formed by the right and left ventricles and the inferior part of the right atrium.

The base (posterior) surface is formed by the right and left atria (Figs. 38 and 39). The four pulmonary veins enter the left atrium at this surface.

The apex is formed by the left ventricle at the fifth intercostal space, approximately 9 cm from the midline.

The cardiac chambers are lined by the endocardium (Fig. 40). The contractile muscular walls of the ventricle are composed of a thicker layer known as the myocardium. The epicardium (or visceral pericardium) is the outer layer of the heart wall.

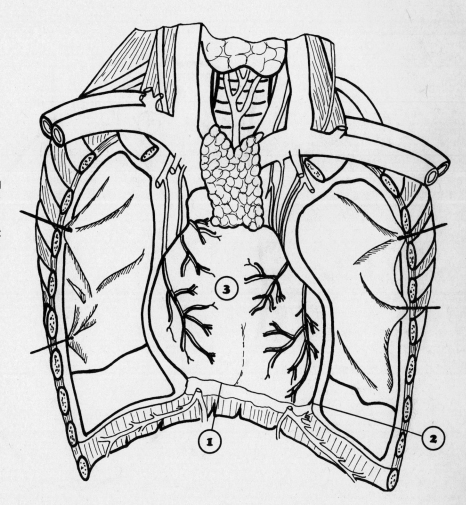

¹Diaphragmatic surface
²Apex
³Sternocostal surface

Fig. 36B ANTERIOR VIEW OF THE HEART

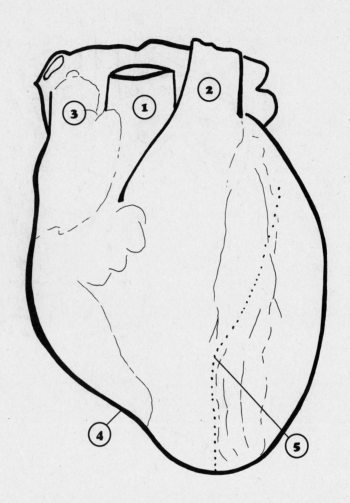

¹Aorta
²Pulmonary trunk
³Superior vena cava
⁴Acute margin
⁵Anterior
   interventricular
   sulcus

Fig. 37 DIAPHRAGMATIC VIEW OF THE HEART (POSTERIOR ASPECT)

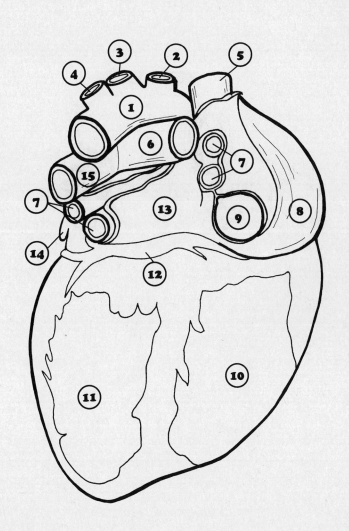

1. Aortic arch
2. Brachiocephalic artery
3. Left common carotid artery
4. Left subclavian artery
5. Superior vena cava
6. Right pulmonary artery
7. Pulmonary vein
8. Right atrium
9. Inferior vena cava
10. Right ventricle
11. Left ventricle
12. Coronary sinus
13. Left atrium
14. Left auricle
15. Left pulmonary artery

Fig. 38 POSTERIOR (BASAL) VIEW OF THE HEART

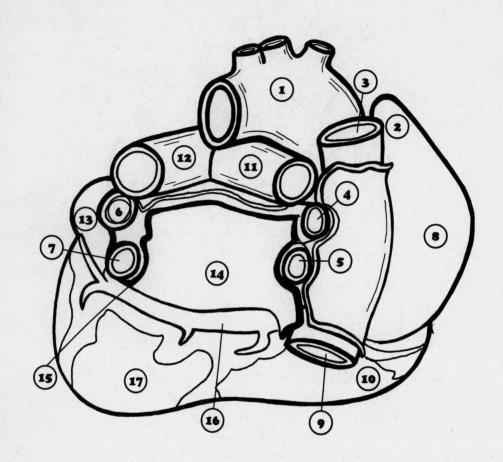

¹Aortic arch
²Right auricle
³Superior vena cava
⁴Right superior
   pulmonary vein
⁵Right inferior
   pulmonary vein
⁶Left superior
   pulmonary vein
⁷Left inferior
   pulmonary vein

⁸Right atrium
⁹Inferior vena cava
¹⁰Right ventricle
¹¹Right pulmonary
   artery
¹²Left pulmonary artery
¹³Left auricle
¹⁴Left atrium
¹⁵Pericardial reflection
¹⁶Coronary sinus
¹⁷Left ventricle

Fig. 39 HEART VIEWED FROM THE BASE WITH THE ATRIA REMOVED

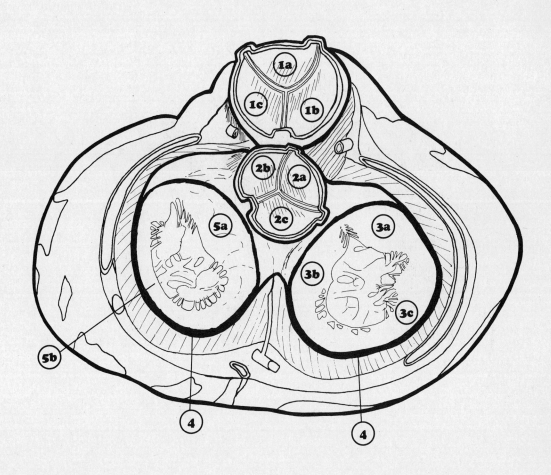

¹Pulmonary valve
¹ᵃAnterior cusp
¹ᵇRight cusp
¹ᶜLeft cusp
²Aortic valve
²ᵃRight coronary cusp
²ᵇLeft coronary cusp
²ᶜNoncoronary cusp

³Tricuspid valve
³ᵃAnterior cusp
³ᵇMedial (septal) cusp
³ᶜPosterior cusp
⁴Annulus fibrosus
⁵Mitral valve
⁵ᵃAnterior cusp
⁵ᵇPosterior cusp

Fig. 40 PARASAGITTAL LONG-AXIS VIEW OF THE HEART

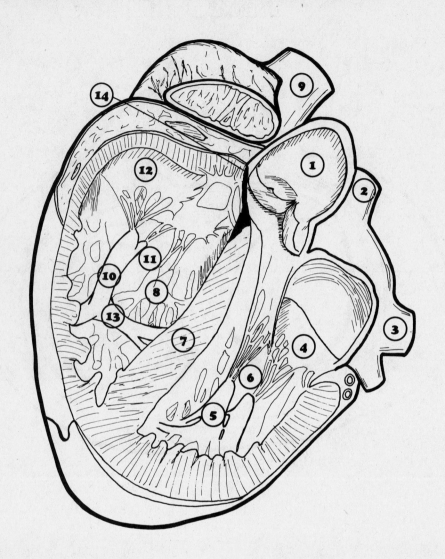

1 Ascending aorta
2 Right pulmonary vein
3 Left pulmonary vein
4 Mitral valve
5 Posterior papillary muscle
6 Left ventricle
7 Muscular interventricular septum

8 Right posterior papillary muscle
9 Superior vena cava
10 Septal band
11 Right ventricle
12 Tricuspid valve
13 Moderator band
14 Membranous interventricular septum

Fig. 41 GREAT VEINS IN THE SUPERIOR MEDIASTINUM

Great Veins in the Superior Mediastinum (Fig. 41)

Brachiocephalic Veins

The right brachiocephalic vein is formed at the root of the neck by the union of the right sub-clavian and right internal jugular veins. The left brachiocephalic vein has a similar origin as it passes obliquely downward and to the right behind the manubrium sterni and in front of the large branches of the aortic arch. It joins the right brachiocephalic vein to form the su-perior vena cava.

Superior Vena Cava

The superior vena cava contains the blood re-turning from the head, neck, and upper ex-tremities. It passes downward to enter the su-perior part of the right atrium of the heart. The vena azygos joins the posterior aspect of the superior vena cava before it enters the peri-cardial sac.

Inferior Vena Cava

The inferior vena cava penetrates the central tendon of the diaphragm to enter the lowest part of the right atrium. It brings blood back from the abdominal organs, pelvis, and lower extremities.

Pulmonary Veins

The four pulmonary veins leave each lung car-rying oxygenated blood to the left atrium of the heart.

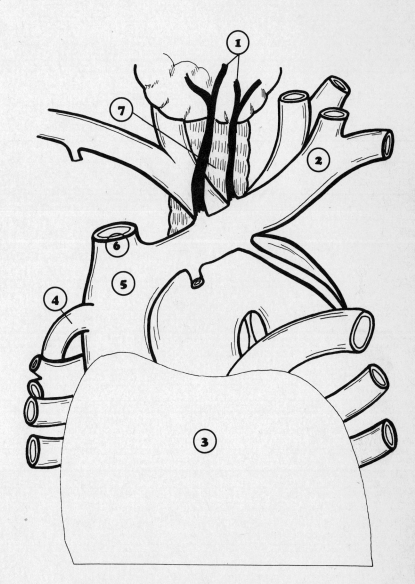

[1] Inferior thyroid veins
[2] Left brachiocephalic vein
[3] Pericardial sac
[4] Azygos vein
[5] Superior vena cava
[6] Right brachiocephalic vein
[7] Trachea

Fig. 42 AORTIC ARCH AND ITS BRANCHES

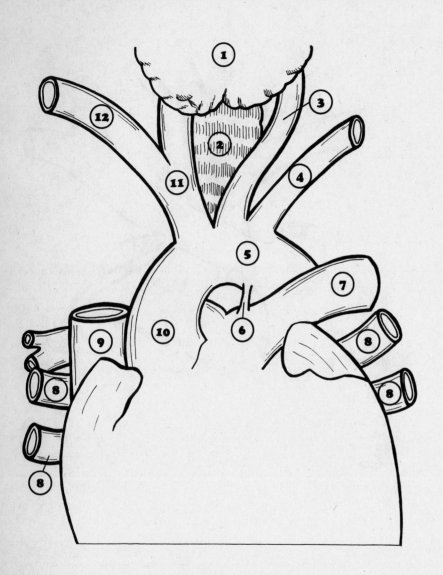

Aortic Arch and Its Branches (Fig. 42)

The aortic arch is a continuation of the ascending aorta. It lies behind the manubrium sterni and runs upward, backward, and to the left in front of the trachea. It then passes downward to the left of the trachea to become continuous with the descending aorta at the sternal angle.

Branches of the Aorta

The brachiocephalic artery arises from the convex surface of the arch. It passes upward and to the right of the trachea and divides into the right subclavian and common carotid arteries.

The left common carotid artery arises from the aortic arch on the left side of the brachiocephalic artery. It runs upward and to the left of the trachea and enters the neck behind the left sternoclavicular joint.

The left subclavian artery arises from the arch behind the left common carotid artery. It runs upward along the right side of the trachea and the esophagus to enter the root of the neck.

Pulmonary Trunk

The pulmonary trunk leaves the right ventricle of the heart and runs upward, backward, and to the left. It terminates in the concavity of the aortic arch by dividing into the right and left pulmonary arteries. Along with the ascending aorta, it is enclosed in a sheath of serous pericardium.

Branches of the Pulmonary Artery

The right pulmonary artery runs to the right behind the ascending aorta and the superior vena cava to enter the root of the right lung.

The left pulmonary artery runs to the left in front of the descending aorta to enter the root of the left lung.

The ligamentum arteriosum is a fibrous band that connects the bifurcation of the pulmonary trunk to the lower surface of the aortic arch. The ligamentum arteriosum is the remains of the ductus arteriosus in the fetus.

¹Thyroid gland
²Trachea
³Left common carotid artery
⁴Left subclavian artery
⁵Aortic arch
⁶Ligamentum arteriosum
⁷Left pulmonary artery
⁸Pulmonary veins
⁹Superior vena cava
¹⁰Ascending aorta
¹¹Brachiocephalic trunk
¹²Right subclavian artery

Fig. 43 PERICARDIUM*

Arrows indicate the pericardial sac.

Pericardium (Fig. 43)

The pericardium is a double sac that encloses the heart and the great vessels. The fibrous pericardium limits the movement of the heart. It is attached inferiorly to the central tendon of the diaphragm. Superiorly it reflects off the roots of the great vessels. Anteriorly it is attached to the sternum by the sternopericardial ligaments.

The serous pericardium is divided into two layers: parietal and visceral. The parietal layer lines the fibrous pericardium and is reflected around the roots of the great vessels, where it becomes continuous with the visceral layer of serous pericardium.

The visceral layer is often called the *epicardium of the heart wall.* The small space between the parietal and visceral layers is the pericardial cavity. This cavity normally contains a small amount of pericardial fluid to help facilitate cardiac movement.

Two sinuses are found on the posterior base of the heart. The oblique sinus is found at the point where the serous pericardium reflects around the large veins. The transverse sinus is a recess that lies between the reflection of the serous pericardium and the great arteries and veins.

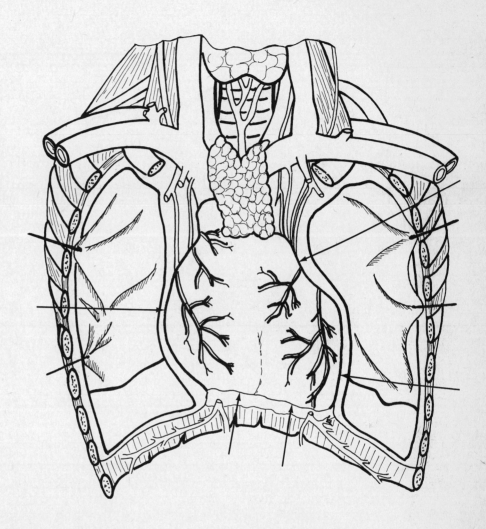

Fig. 44 RIGHT ATRIUM VIEWED FROM THE RIGHT SIDE

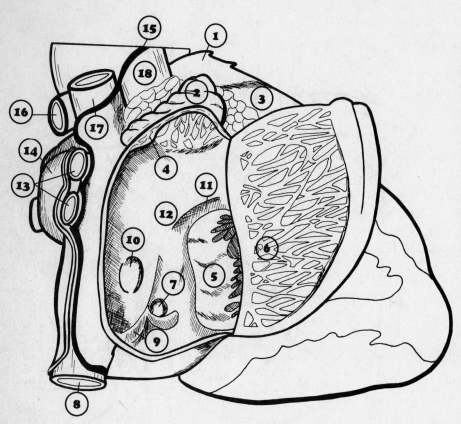

Right Atrium and Interatrial Septum (Fig. 44)

The right atrium forms the right border of the heart. The superior vena cava enters the upper posterior border, and the inferior vena cava enters the lower posterior border. The pulmonary veins travel posterior to the right atrial wall.

The interior of the atrium is separated into two parts by a ridge of muscle, the crista terminalis. The posterior part of the atrium is very smooth walled, probably owing to the continual flow of blood from the interior and superior venae cavae and the coronary sinus. The inferior vena cava is guarded by a fold of tissue called the eustachian valve, while the coronary sinus is guarded by the thebesian valve. The atrium anterior to the ridge is trabeculated by muscle bundles known as pectinate muscles. The right atrial appendage (the most superior portion) contains the most prominent pectinate muscles.

The posterior medial wall of the right atrium is formed by the atrial septum. The central portion of the septum is thin and fibrous. The fossa ovalis, the site of the formen ovale in the fetus, is the shallow depression just superior and anterior to the inferior vena cava. Its borders are the limbus fossae ovalis and the primitive septum primum. The tricuspid valve annulus is formed from the lower edge of the septum secundum.

The coronary sinus drains the blood supply from the heart wall. It is bordered by the fossa ovalis and the tricuspid valve.

The right atrioventricular orifice is guarded by the tricuspid valve.

¹Pulmonary trunk
²Right auricle
³Conus arteriosus
⁴Crista terminalis
⁵Medial cusp of the tricuspid valve
⁶Pectinate muscles
⁷Orifice of the coronary sinus
⁸Inferior vena cava
⁹Eustachian valve
¹⁰Fossa ovalis
¹¹Membranous septum
¹²Interatrial septum
¹³Right inferior and superior pulmonary veins
¹⁴Left atrium
¹⁵Pericardial reflection
¹⁶Right pulmonary artery
¹⁷Superior vena cava
¹⁸Aorta

Fig. 45 TRICUSPID VALVE

Tricuspid Valve (Fig. 45)

The tricuspid valve has three leaflets: anterior, septal, and inferior (or mural). Each leaflet has a double layer of endocardium with a small amount of fibrous tissue. The leaflets are attached by their bases to the atrioventricular ring. The chordae tendineae attach the leaflets to the papillary muscles. When the ventricle contracts, the papillary muscles contract, pull the leaflets together, and prevent them from being forced backward into the atrial cavity as ventricular pressure rises. The chordae tendineae assist in this process; they are attached to both leaflets and papillary muscles to prevent leaflet "sagging" during systole.

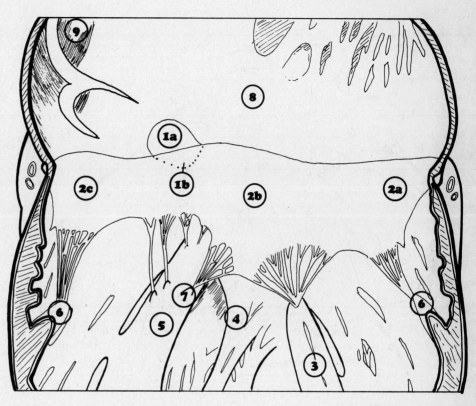

¹Membranous septum
¹ᵃAtrioventricular part
¹ᵇInterventricular part
 (behind valve)
²Tricuspid valve
²ᵃPosterior cusp
²ᵇAnterior cusp
²ᶜMedial cusp
³Anterior papillary
 muscle

⁴Parietal band
⁵Septal band
⁶Posterior papillary
 muscles (sectioned)
⁷Medial (conal) papillary
 muscle
⁸Right atrium
⁹Inferior vena cava

Fig. 46 ANTERIOR VIEW OF THE RIGHT VENTRICLE

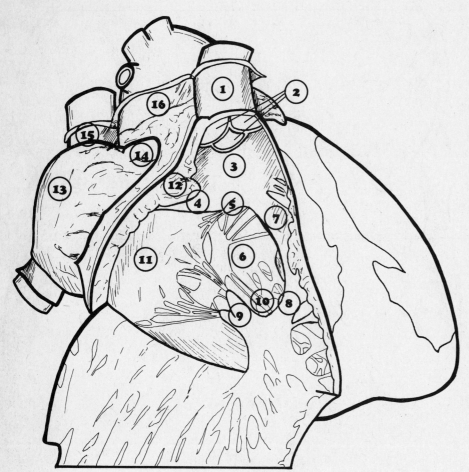

Right Ventricle (Fig. 46)

The base of the right ventricle rests on the diaphragm. The "roof" of the ventricle, (which lies between the pulmonary and tricuspid orifices,) is known as the supraventricular crest.

The right ventricle is divided into two parts: the posteroinferior-inflow portion (containing the tricuspid valve) and the anterosuperior-outflow portion (containing the origin of the pulmonary trunk). These two parts are demarcated by three prominent bands: the parietal band, the septal band, and moderator band (along with the supraventricular crest). The moderator band conveys the right branch of the atrioventricular bundle.

The walls of the right ventricle are thick, irregular ridges of muscle bundles called trabeculae carneae. Some of these trabeculations give rise to the papillary muscle formation.

The inflow tract of the right ventricle is short and very trabeculated. This trabeculated zone is known as the body of the right ventricle.

The inflow tract merges with the outflow tract, or infundibulum. The funnel-shaped outflow tract is smooth walled and contains few trabeculae.

1. Pulmonary trunk
2. Pulmonary valve
3. Conus arteriosus
4. Supraventricular crest
5. Medial papillary muscle
6. Interventricular septum
7. Septal band
8. Moderator band
9. Anterior papillary muscle
10. Posterior papillary muscle
11. Tricuspid valve
12. Parietal band
13. Right atrium
14. Right auricle
15. Superior vena cava
16. Aorta

Fig. 47 CORONAL SECTION THROUGH THE THORAX IN A PLANE SLIGHTLY IN FRONT OF THE MIDAXILLARY LINES

Pulmonary Valve

The pulmonary valve lies at the anterior aspect of the right ventricle (Fig. 47). It has three semilunar cusps: anterior, right, and left. The cusps are composed of a double layer of endocardium and a small amount of fibrous tissue. The lower borders of each cusp are curved and are attached to the pulmonary arterial wall. The open mouth or "pocket" of each cusp faces upward. These dilatations are called sinuses.

The main pulmonary artery projects posterior and slightly upward from the right ventricle to bifurcate into the right and left pulmonary arteries. The ligamentum arteriosum, a remnant of the fetal ductus arteriosus, connects the upper aspect of the bifucation to the anterior surface of the aortic arch.

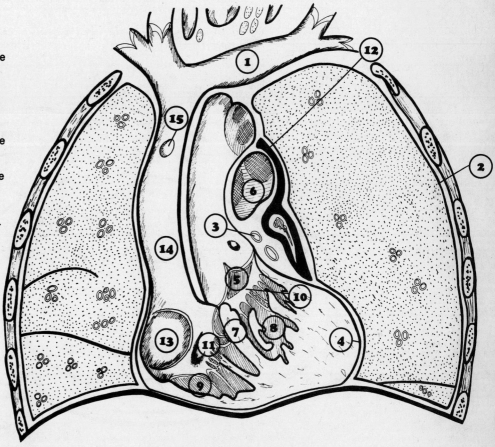

¹Left brachiocephalic vein
²Parietal pleura
³Coronary sinus
⁴Epicardium
⁵Ascending aorta
⁶Pulmonary artery
⁷Interventricular septum
⁸Left ventricle
⁹Right ventricle
¹⁰Mitral valve
¹¹Tricuspid valve
¹²Pericardial sac
¹³Ostium of the inferior vena cava
¹⁴Superior vena cava
¹⁵Azygos vein (ostium)

Fig. 48 POSTEROLATERAL VIEW OF THE LEFT ATRIUM AND VENTRICLE

Left Atrium (Fig. 48)

The left atrium is posterior to the right atrium and forms the greater surface of the base of the heart. The oblique sinus of the serous pericardium lies posterior, and it is separated from the esophagus by the fibrous pericardium.

The atrium is smooth walled, except for its small, pectinated atrial appendage. Two pulmonary veins from each lung open into its posterior wall.

The septal surface of the atrium is fairly smooth, except for the site of the remnant valve of the foramen ovalae.

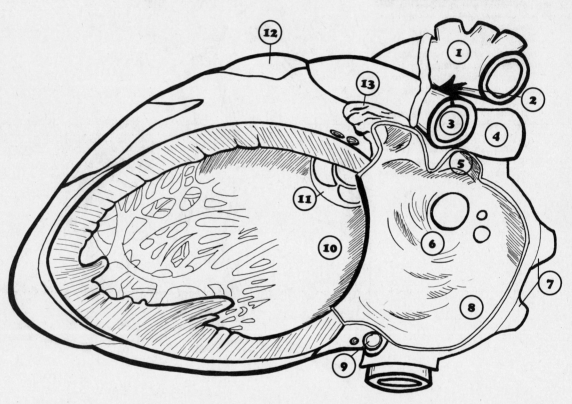

¹Aortic arch
²Ligamentum arteriosum
³Left pulmonary artery
⁴Right pulmonary artery
⁵Left superior pulmonary vein
⁶Valve of the foramen ovale
⁷Right pulmonary veins
⁸Left atrium
⁹Coronary sinus
¹⁰Mitral valve (cut away)
¹¹Aortic valve
¹²Conus arteriosus
¹³Left auricle

Fig. 49 MITRAL VALVE

Mitral Valve (Fig. 49)

The mitral valve separates the left atrium from the left ventricle. It has two basic leaflets. The anterior leaflet is much larger and longer than the posterior leaflet, each of which is attached at its base to the mitral annulus. The chordae tendineae attach the tips of the leaflets to the papillary muscles and serve the same function as in the tricuspid valve.

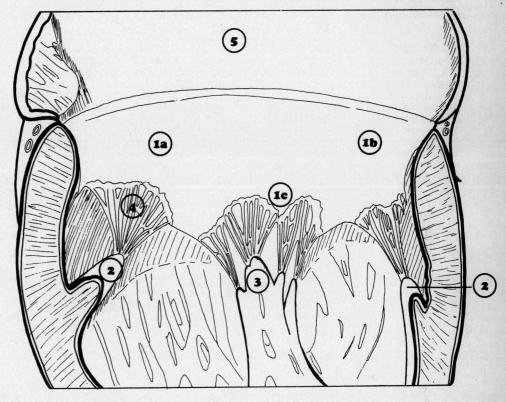

[1] Mitral valve
[1a] Anterior cusp
[1b] Posterior cusp
[1c] Commissural cusps
[2] Anterior papillary muscle
[3] Posterior papillary muscle
[4] Chordae tendineae
[5] Left atrium

Fig. 50 POSTEROLATERAL VIEW OF THE LEFT VENTRICLE

Left Ventricle and Interventricular Septum (Fig. 50)

The elipsoid left ventricle has a short inflow tract that extends from the mitral valve to the trabecular zone. This inflow tract merges with the outflow tract, which extends to the base of the aortic valve.

The smallest and most inferior end of the ventricle is the apex. The larger end, near the aorta and mitral valve, is called the base.

The anterior leaflet of the mitral valve is continuous with the posterior aortic wall, and the interventricular septum is continuous with the anterior aortic wall.

The medial wall of the left ventricle is formed by the ventricular septum. The septum is separated into four parts: membranous, inflow, trabecular, and infundibular. The thinnest part of the septum is the membranous section, located just inferior to the junction of the interatrial septum and the aortic root.

The majority of the septum is muscular. It consists of two layers: a thin layer on the right and a thicker layer on the left. The major septal coronary arteries run between these layers. The muscular part of the septum has approximately the same thickness as the posterior left

ventricular wall. The left ventricular wall is generally two to three times the thickness of the right ventricular wall. Three layers constitute the ventricular wall: the thin, inner layer (endocardium), the thick, middle layer (myocardium), and the outer layer (epicardium, visceral pericardium).

The lateral wall of the left ventricle is covered with fine, numerous strands of trabeculae.

The upper posterior part of the left ventricular wall below the aortic-outflow tract is relatively smooth and is termed the aortic vestibule.

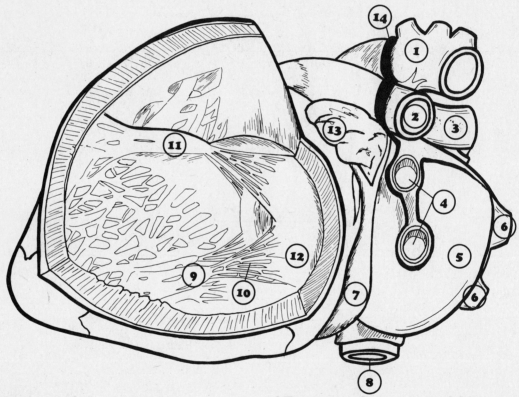

¹Aortic arch
²Left pulmonary artery
³Right pulmonary artery
⁴Left pulmonary veins
⁵Left atrium
⁶Right pulmonary veins
⁷Coronary sinus
⁸Inferior vena cava
⁹Posterior papillary muscle
¹⁰Chordae tendineae
¹¹Anterior papillary muscle
¹²Mitral valve
¹³Left auricle
¹⁴Pericardial reflection

Fig. 51 AORTIC VALVE

Aortic Valve (Fig. 51)

The aortic valve lies at the root of the ascending aorta at the base of the heart. Like the pulmonary valve, it has three semilunar cusps: the right coronary, the noncoronary (posterior), and the left coronary. A sinus of Valsalva is found at the base of each cusp. During ventricular systole, the cusps of the valve are pressed open by the pressure of blood flow. During diastole, blood flows backward to fill the sinuses and close the cusps. At the center of each cusp is a small fibrous nodule, Arantius's nodule, which aids the cusps in preventing blood leakage when it closes.

The two coronary arteries arise from the right and left coronary cusps.

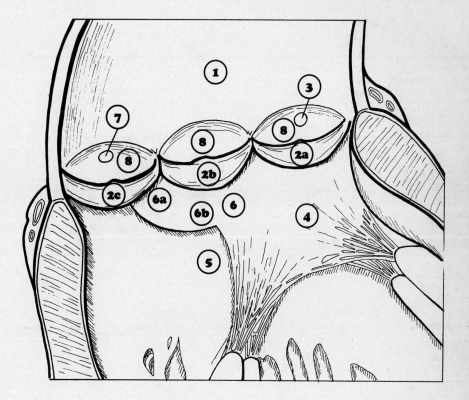

¹Ascending aorta
²Aortic valve
²ᵃLeft cusp
²ᵇPosterior cusp
²ᶜRight cusp
³Orifice of the left coronary artery
⁴Anterior mitral valve leaflet

⁵Muscular interventricular septum
⁶Membranous septum
⁶ᵃInterventricular part
⁶ᵇAtrioventricular part
⁷Orifice of the right coronary artery
⁸Aortic sinuses of Valsalva

Fig. 52 CONDUCTING SYSTEM OF THE HEART

CARDIAC CYCLE AND THE CONDUCTING SYSTEM OF THE HEART

The heart is a muscular pump that propels blood to all parts of the body. The cardiac cycle is the series of changes that the heart undergoes as it fills with blood and empties. The rhythmic contraction of the heart causes the blood to be pumped through the chambers of the heart and out through the great vessels to the rest of the body. The forceful contraction of the cardiac chambers is called systole. The relaxed phase of the cycle is diastole.

During diastole the venous blood enters the right atrium from the superior and inferior venae cavae. At the same time, the oxygenated blood returns from the lungs through the pulmonary veins to enter the left atrium. The atrioventricular valves (tricuspid and mitral) between the atria and ventricles are open so the blood may flow from the atria into the ventricles. In the next phase, atrial contraction squeezes the remaining blood from the atria

into the ventricles. The combination of atrial contraction and increased pressure of the full atrial cavities ultimately drains the atrial blood into the ventricles. Shortly after this phase, the ventricles contract (called ventricular systole). The rising pressure in the ventricular cavity closes the atrioventricular valves. As the pressure increases in the ventricles, the semilunar valves (pulmonary and aortic) open so that blood can be forced into the lungs and body, respectively.

The ventricles relax when contraction is completed (called ventricular diastole). The blood in the aorta is under very high pressure, and the decreased pressure in the ventricles could cause it to flow backward into the ventricles. However, the semilunar valves prevent this reverse flow. The blood fills the sinuses of Valsalva and forces the valves to close. During ventricular contraction, the atria relax, and the venous blood starts to fill the atria again. When the ventricles are completely relaxed, the atrioventricular valves open, and blood flows into the ventricles to begin the next cardiac cycle.

The conducting system of the heart consists of specialized cardiac muscle in the sinoatrial node, the atrioventricular node, the atrioventricular bundle and its right and left terminal branches, and the subendocardial plexus of Purkinje fibers (Fig. 52). The sinoatrial node is the location where the contraction of the heart muscle is initiated and is often called the pacemaker. It is situated in the right atrium, at the upper part of the sulcus terminalis just to the right of the opening of the superior vena cava. Once activated, the cardiac impulse spreads through the atrial myocardium to reach the atrioventricular node.

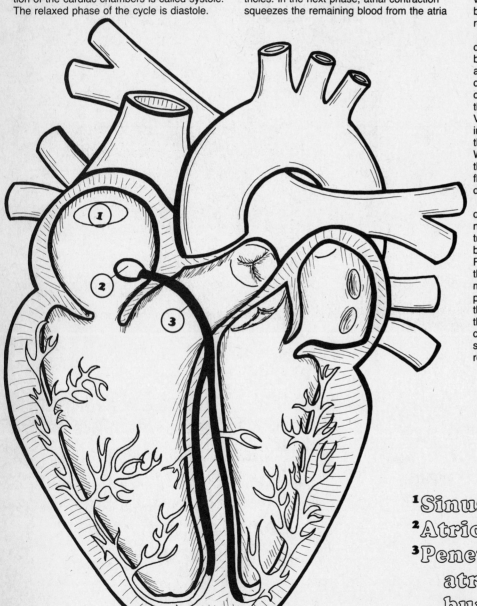

¹Sinus node
²Atrioventricular node
³Penetrating atrioventricular bundle (bundle of His)
⁴Purkinje fibers

54

Fig. 53 THORACIC CROSS SECTION, LEVEL 1

The atrioventricular node is located in the lower part of the atrial septum just above the attachment of the septal cusp of the tricuspid valve. The cardiac impulse is further transmitted to the ventricles by the atrioventricular bundle.

The atrioventricular bundle descends behind the septal leaflet of the tricuspid valve to reach the inferior border of the membranous part of the ventricular septum. It divides into two branches at the upper border of the muscular part of the septum. The right branch passes along the right side of the septum to touch the moderator band in the right ventricle. It crosses to the anterior wall of the right ventricle by the moderator band to become continuous with the fibers of the Purkinje plexus.

The left branch of the bundle pierces the septum and passes down beneath the endocardium. It divides into the branches that eventually become continuous with the fibers of the Purkinje plexus of the left ventricle.

SERIAL THORACIC CROSS SECTIONS

Thoracic Cross Section, Level 1 (Fig. 53)

This section is taken at the level of the fourth thoracic vertebra. The aortic arch is cut along its lower border. The ascending and descending aorta is shown in part. The right and left pulmonary arteries originate in the lower portion of this section. The superior vena cava is shown as it enters the right atrium. The pericardium is reflected to show a portion of the pericardial cavity. The trachea is shown to the right of the mesial plane. The bronchi begin to subdivide in the body of this section.

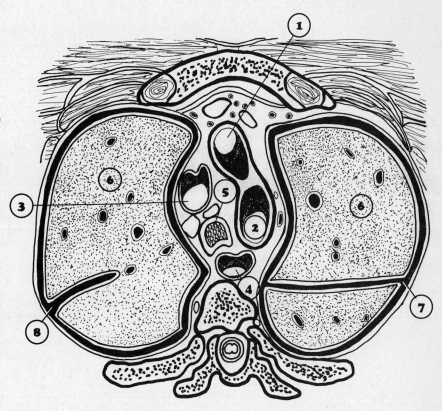

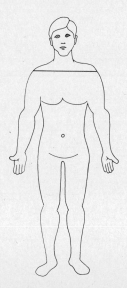

¹Ascending aorta
²Descending aorta
³Superior vena cava
⁴Esophagus
⁵Trachea
⁶Superior lobe of the lung
⁷Interlobar incisure
⁸Accessory incisure

Fig. 54 THORACIC CROSS SECTION, LEVEL 2

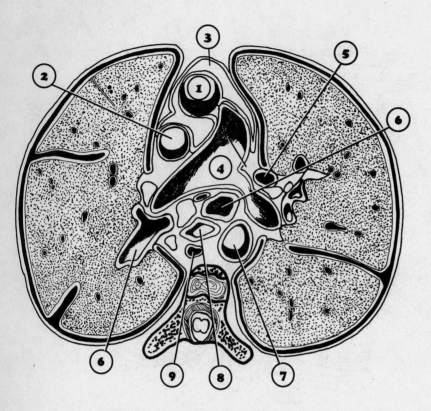

Thoracic Cross Section, Level 2 (Fig. 54)

This section is taken at the level of the fifth thoracic disc. The ascending and descending parts of the aorta are shown. The superior vena cava enters the right atrium in the lower portion of this section and the upper portion of Level 1. The pulmonary valves are shown in the pulmonary artery. The atrial appendages are seen within this section, as is the conus arteriosus. The trachea has bifurcated, and the bronchi are seen. The esophagus lies in the midline.

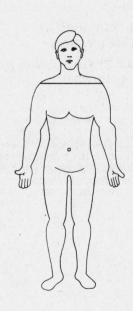

¹Ascending aorta
²Superior vena cava
³Conus arteriosus
⁴Pulmonary artery
⁵Pulmonary vein
⁶Bronchus
⁷Thoracic aorta
⁸Esophagus
⁹Azygos vein

Fig. 55 THORACIC CROSS SECTION, LEVEL 3

Thoracic Cross Section, Level 3 (Fig. 55)

This section is taken at the upper part of the seventh thoracic vertebra. The right atrium is shown at the entrance of the superior vena cava. The left atrium is shown just below the entrance of the right superior pulmonary vein. The right inferior pulmonary vein enters the atrium within this section. The left superior pulmonary vein is cut at its entrance into the left atrium. The left inferior pulmonary vein enters the left atrium within this section. The fo-ramen ovale is slightly open in the interatrial septum. The aortic valve and the sinuses of Valsalva are shown. The right ventricle shows the cordae tendineae, which are attached to the tricuspid leaflets. The pulmonary valve lies anterior to and to the left of the aortic valve. The mitral valve lies partly in this section and partly in Level 2. The right coronary artery is shown as it arises from the right coronary cusp.

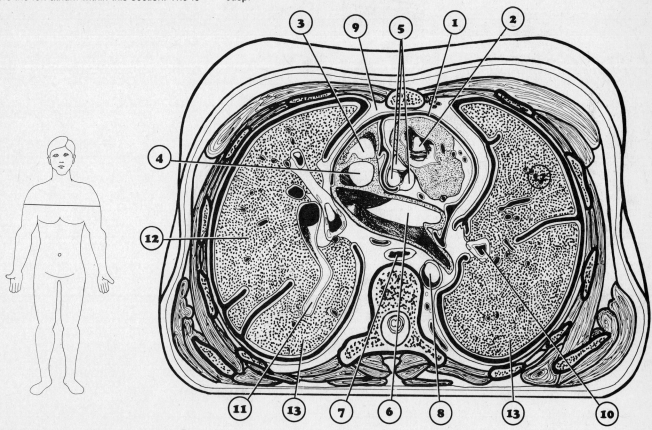

¹Pericardial sac
²Right ventricle, chordae tendineae
³Right atrium
⁴Superior vena cava
⁵Aortic valve
⁶Left atrium
⁷Esophagus
⁸Descending aorta
⁹Anterior mediastinum
¹⁰Bronchus
¹¹Right pulmonary vein
¹²Superior lobe of the lung
¹³Inferior lobe of the lung

Fig. 56 THORACIC CROSS SECTION, LEVEL 4

Thoracic Cross Section, Level 4 (Fig. 56)

This section is taken at the level of the eighth thoracic vertebra. The diaphragm extends into the lower portion of this section, and the right and left atria and ventricles are shown, as is the opening of the inferior vena cava into the right atrium. The eustachian valve of the orifice of the inferior vena cava can be seen. The tricuspid valve and mitral valve are both shown as they separate the atria from the ventricular chambers. The coronary sinus opens into the right atrium at the arrow. The esophagus is shown slightly to the left of midline.

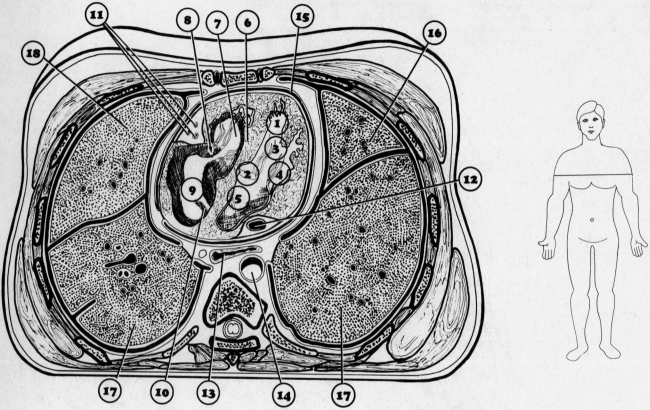

¹Left ventricle
²Anterior leaflet of the mitral valve
³Chordae tendineae
⁴Posterior leaflet of the mitral valve
⁵Left atrium
⁶Interventricular septum
⁷Right ventricle
⁸Tricuspid valve
⁹Right atrium

¹⁰Eustachian valve (to the inferior vena cava)
¹¹Right coronary artery
¹²Coronary sinus
¹³Esophagus
¹⁴Descending aorta
¹⁵Pericardial sac
¹⁶Superior lobe of the lung
¹⁷Inferior lobe of the lung
¹⁸Medial lobe of the lung

Fig. 57 THORACIC CROSS SECTION, LEVEL 5

Thoracic Cross Section, Level 5 (Fig. 57)

This section is taken at the level of the ninth intervertebral disc. The pleural surface of the diaphragm is seen on the right. On the left, oblique fibers of the diaphragm are shown. The right atrium and left ventricles are seen. The pericardium, epicardium, and pericardial cavity are shown. The hepatic vein is shown to enter the inferior vena cava at the level of the diaphragm.

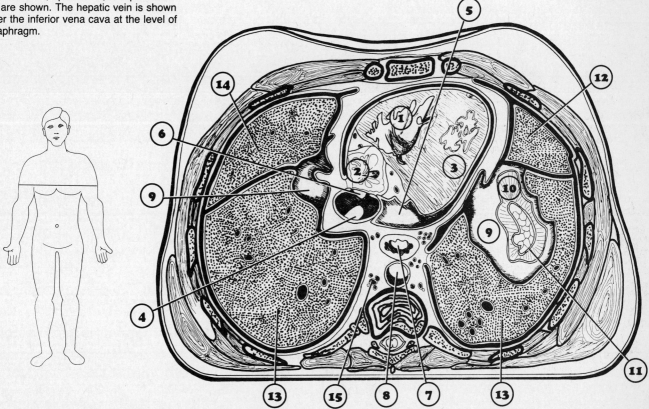

[1] Right ventricle
[2] Right atrium
[3] Left ventricle
[4] Inferior vena cava
[5] Pericardial sac
[6] Hepatic vein
[7] Esophagus
[8] Descending aorta
[9] Diaphragmatic pleura
[10] Diaphragm
[11] Parietal peritoneum
[12] Superior lobe of the lung
[13] Inferior lobe of the lung
[14] Medial lobe of the lung
[15] Azygos vein

Fetal Circulation

Fig. 58 *IN UTERO FETAL CIRCULATION*

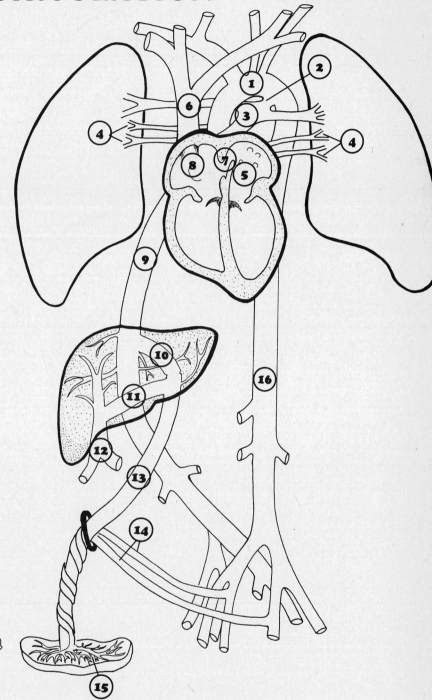

BEFORE BIRTH (Fig. 58)

Oxygenated blood returns via the umbilical vein from the placenta to the heart. Approximately half of the blood passes through the hepatic sinusoids, while the rest bypasses the liver to go through the ductus venosus into the inferior vena cava.

The blood then enters the right atrium after a short course in the inferior vena cava. The blood in the right atrium is less oxygenated than the blood in the umbilical vein. The blood from the inferior vena cava is directed by the lower border of the septum secundum (the crista dividens) through the foramen ovale into the left atrium. It mixes with a small amount of deoxygenated blood returning from the lungs via the pulmonary veins into the left atrium. The blood then flows into the left ventricle and leaves through the ascending aorta.

A small amount of oxygenated blood from the inferior vena cava is diverted by the crista dividens and remains in the right atrium to mix with deoxygenated blood from the superior vena cava and coronary sinus. This blood flows into the right ventricle and leaves via the pulmonary artery. Most of the blood passes through the patent ductus arteriosus into the aorta. Only a very small amount goes to the lungs. Most of the mixed blood in the descending aorta passes into the umbilical arteries and is returned to the placenta for reoxygenation. The remainder of the blood circulates through the lower part of the body.

1 Aortic arch
2 Ductus arteriosus
3 Pulmonary trunk
4 Pulmonary veins
5 Left atrium
6 Superior vena cava
7 Foramen ovale
8 Right atrium
9 Inferior vena cava
10 Ductus venosus
11 Portal sinus
12 Portal vein
13 Umbilical vein
14 Umbilical arteries
15 Placenta
16 Descending aorta

Fig. 59 NEONATAL CIRCULATION

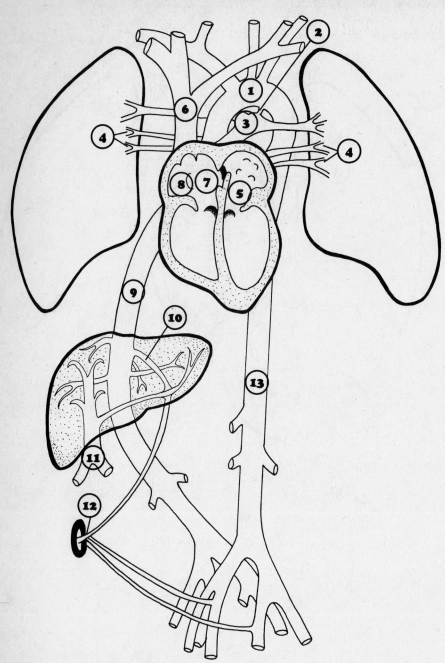

AFTER BIRTH (Fig. 59)

After birth, the circulation of the fetal blood through the placenta ceases, and the newborn's lungs begin to function. The fetal cardiac structures that are no longer needed are the foramen ovale, the ductus arteriosus, the ductus venosus, and the umbilical vessels. Omission of the placental circulation causes an immediate fall of blood pressure in the newborn's inferior vena cava and right atrium. As the lungs aerate, there is a fall in the pulmonary vascular resistance. This causes an increase in pulmonary blood flow and a progressive thinning of the walls of the pulmonary arteries. Thus the pressure in the left atrium becomes higher than that in the right atrium. This causes the foramen ovale to close (the foramen opens into the left atrial cavity in the fetus) by pressing its valve (the septum primum) against the septum secundum.

The ductus arteriosus usually constricts shortly after birth, once the left-sided pressures exceed the right-sided pressures. Often, there is a small shunt of blood from the aorta to the pulmonary artery until these pressures adjust to neonatal life.

The umbilical arteries likewise constrict after birth to prevent blood loss from the infant.

ADULT DERIVATIVES OF FETAL VESSELS AND STRUCTURES

As noted previously, certain vessels and other structures are not necessary after birth of the fetus. Others persist into adulthood. The intra-abdominal portion of the umbilical vein forms the ligamentum teres. This structure passes from the umbilicus to the porta hepatis, where it attaches to the left branch of the portal vein.

The umbilical vein may remain patent for some time after birth.

The ductus venosus becomes the ligamentum venosum. This structure passes through the liver from the left branch of the portal vein to the inferior vena cava.

The abdominal portions of the umbilical arteries form the lateral umbilical ligaments. The proximal parts of these vessels are the superior vesical arteries.

The foramen ovale usually closes shortly after birth. With time, complete closure occurs from adhesion of the septum primum to the left margin of the septum secundum. The septum primum forms the floor of the fossa ovalis. The lower edge of the septum secundum forms the limbus fossae ovalis, which demarcates the former cranial boundary of the foramen ovale.

The ductus arteriosus turns into the ligamentum arteriosum. This structure passes from the left pulmonary artery to the arch of the aorta.

1. Aortic arch
2. Ligamentum arteriosum
3. Pulmonary trunk
4. Pulmonary veins
5. Left atrium
6. Superior vena cava
7. Foramen ovale (closed)
8. Right atrium
9. Inferior vena cava
10. Ligamentum venosum
11. Portal vein
12. Ligamentum teres
13. Descending aorta

The Abdomen in General

Fig. 60 SURFACE LANDMARKS OF THE ANTERIOR ABDOMINAL WALL

SURFACE LANDMARKS

Xyphoid process (Fig. 60) Half as thick as the sternum and easily palpated in the depression where the costal margins meet at the infrasternal angle

Costal margin The curved lower margin of the thoracic wall. It is formed anteriorly by the cartilages of the seventh, eighth, ninth, and tenth ribs and posteriorly by the eleventh and twelfth ribs. Its lowest level is at the tenth rib, which lies opposite the body of the third lumbar vertebra.

Iliac crest (Fig. 61) May be easily palpated and ends in front at the anterior iliac spine and behind at the posterior iliac spine. Its highest point lies opposite the body of the fourth lumbar vertebra.

Inguinal ligament The rolled inferior margin of the aponeurosis of the external oblique muscle. It is attached laterally to the anterior superior iliac spine and curves downward and medial to the pubic tubercle.

Pubic tubercle A small protuberance along the superior surface of the pubis

Pubic symphysis A cartilaginous joint that lies in the midline between the bodies of the pubic bones

Mid-inguinal point A point that lies on the inguinal ligament halfway between the pubic symphysis and the anterior superior iliac spine

Superficial inguinal ring A triangular aperture in the aponeurosis of the external oblique muscle situated above and medial to the pubic tubercle

Linea alba A midline fibrous band that extends from the pubic symphysis to the xyphoid process. It is formed by the fusion of the aponeuroses of the anterior abdominal wall muscles and is revealed on the surface by a slight median groove.

Umbilicus The remnant of the fetal umbilical cord. It lies in the linea alba and varies in position.

Linea semilunaris (Fig. 60) The lateral edge of the rectus abdominis muscle.

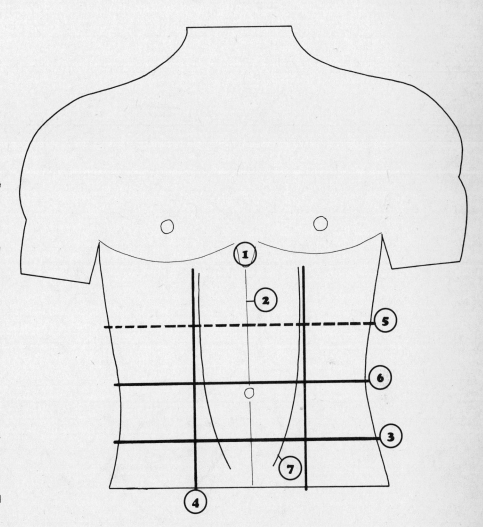

¹Xyphoid process
²Median groove
³Tubercle of crest (intertubercular plane)
⁴Right lateral plane
⁵Transpyloric plane
⁶Subcostal plane
⁷Linea semilunaris

Fig. 61 LANDMARKS OF THE POSTERIOR TORSO

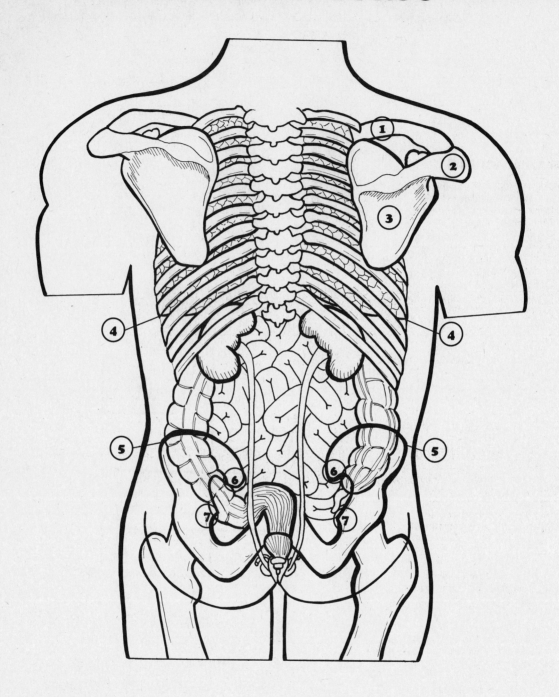

¹Clavicle
²Acromion
³Scapula
⁴Costodiaphragmatic
   recess

⁵Iliac crest
⁶Posterior superior iliac
   spine
⁷Ischial spine

Fig. 62 REGIONS OF THE ABDOMINAL WALL

ABDOMINAL REGIONS

The abdomen can be divided into nine regions by two vertical and two horizontal lines (Fig. 62). Each vertical line passes through the mid-inguinal point. The subcostal plane (of the upper horizontal line) joins the lowest point of the costal margin at the tenth costal cartilage and lies opposite the third lumbar vertebra. The intertubercular plane (of the lowest horizontal line) joins the tubercles on the iliac crests at the body of the fifth lumbar vertebra.

Upper abdomen
   Right hypochondrium
   Epigastrium
   Left hypochondrium
Middle abdomen
   Right lumbar
   Umbilical
   Left lumbar
Lower abdomen
   Right iliac fossa
   Hypogastrium
   Left iliac fossa

The transpyloric plane passes through the tips of the ninth costal cartilages on both sides. This is the point where the lateral edge of the rectus abdominis (linea semilunaris) crosses the costal margin. This plane passes through the renal hila, the neck of the pancreas, the duodenojejunal junction, and the pylorus.

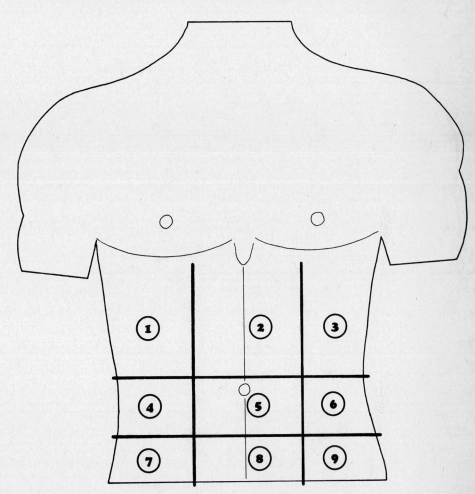

[1] Right hypochondrium
[2] Epigastrium
[3] Left hypochondrium
[4] Right lumbar region
[5] Umbilical region
[6] Left lumbar region
[7] Right iliac fossa
[8] Hypogastrium
[9] Left iliac fossa

Fig. 63 BASIC ABDOMINAL LANDMARKS AND VISCERA

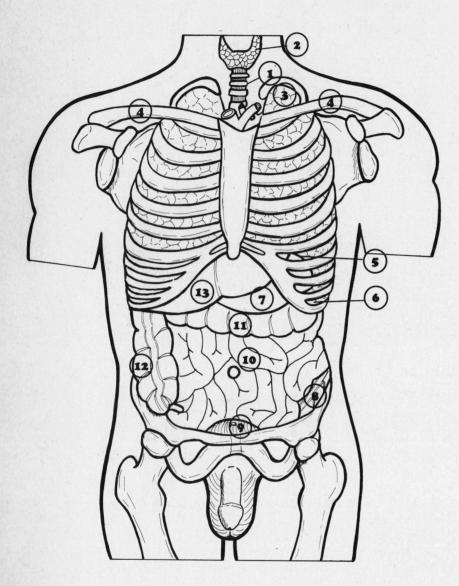

ABDOMINAL CAVITY (Fig. 63)

The abdominal cavity (excluding the retroperitoneum and pelvis) is bounded superiorly by the diaphragm, anteriorly by the abdominal wall muscles, posteriorly by the vertebral column, ribs, and iliac fossa, and inferiorly by the pelvis.

Peritoneum

The peritoneum is a thin, translucent, serous membrane that lines the walls of the abdominal cavity and covers the abdominal viscera. It has two layers: the parietal layer and the visceral layer. The parietal layer lines the walls of the abdominal cavity; the visceral layer covers the abdominal organs. Between the two layers is the peritoneal cavity, which contains a small amount of lubricating serous fluid to permit free movement between the viscera. In the male this cavity is closed, but in the female there is a communication with the exterior through the fallopian tubes, the uterus, and the vagina.

The peritoneal cavity may be divided into two parts: the greater sac and the lesser sac. The greater sac is the larger of the two and extends across the abdomen from the diaphragm to the pelvis. The lesser sac lies posterior to the stomach; as a small diverticulum from the greater sac, it opens through a window called the epiploic foramen.

The mesentery is a two-layered fold of peritoneum that attaches part of the intestine to the posterior abdominal wall, including the small intestine, the transverse colon, and the sigmoid colon.

¹Trachea
²Thyroid
³Pulmonary apex
⁴Clavicle
⁵Diaphragm
⁶Costodiaphragmatic recess

⁷Stomach
⁸Descending colon
⁹Bladder
¹⁰Intestine
¹¹Transverse colon
¹²Ascending colon
¹³Liver

Fig. 64 ABDOMINAL CAVITY

Greater Omentum (Fig. 64)

The omentum is a two-layered fold of peritoneum that attaches the stomach to another viscera. The greater omentum is often referred to as an apron hanging between the small intestine and the anterior abdominal wall and is attached to the greater curvature of the stomach. The lesser omentum attaches the lesser curvature of the stomach to the under-surface of the liver. The gastrosplenic omentum attaches the stomach to the spleen.

There are several peritoneal ligaments that attach the less mobile solid viscera to the abdominal walls:

Falciform ligament: attaches the liver to the abdominal wall and the diaphragm (Fig. 65)

Median umbilical ligament (urachus): passes from the apex of the bladder to the umbilicus

Lateral umbilical ligament: obliterated umbilical arteries, passing from the internal iliac artery to the umbilicus

Ligamentum teres: obliterated umbilical fetal vein, passing upward to enter the groove between the quadrate lobe and the left lobe of the liver

Lienorenal ligament: a peritoneal layer from the kidney to the hilum of the spleen

Gastrosplenic ligament: passes from the hilus of the spleen to the greater curvature of the stomach

The mesenteries, omenta, and peritoneal ligaments allow the blood vessels, lymphatics, and nerves to reach the other viscera in the abdomen (Fig. 66).

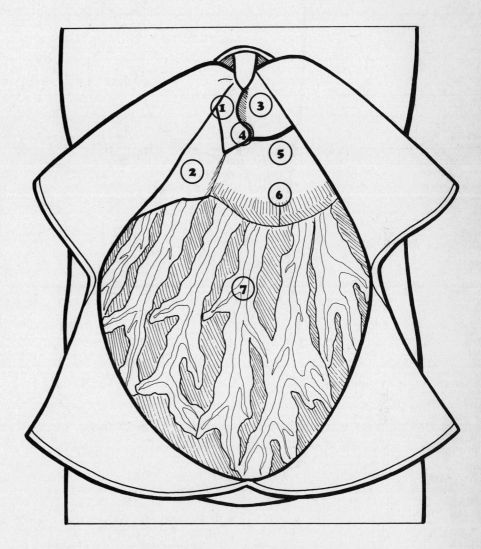

¹Falciform ligament
²Right lobe of the liver
³Left lobe of the liver
⁴Ligamentum teres
⁵Stomach
⁶Greater curvature of the stomach
⁷Greater omentum

Fig. 65 ABDOMINAL CAVITY
(GREATER OMENTUM REMOVED)

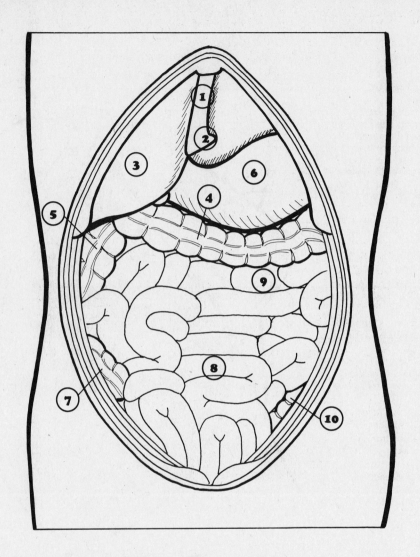

¹Falciform ligament
²Ligamentum teres
³Right lobe of the liver
⁴Transverse colon
⁵Ascending colon
⁶Stomach
⁷Cecum
⁸Ileum
⁹Jejunum
¹⁰Descending colon

Fig.66 TRANSVERSE SECTION OF THE ABDOMINAL CAVITY SHOWING THE REFLECTIONS OF THE PERITONEUM

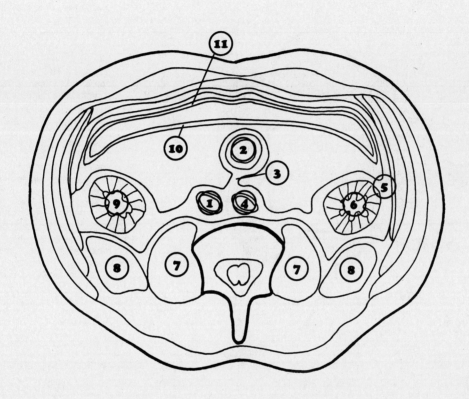

¹Inferior vena cava
²Small intestine
³Mesentery of the small intestine
⁴Aorta
⁵Peritoneum
⁶Descending colon
⁷Psoas major muscle
⁸Quadratus lumborum muscle

⁹Ascending colon
¹⁰Posterior layers of the greater omentum*
¹¹Anterior layers of the greater omentum*

*There is generally no space between the anterior and posterior layers of the greater omentum; they are usually fused together.

Fig. 67A ANTERIOR VIEW OF THE ABDOMINAL VISCERA (LIVER PULLED UPWARD)

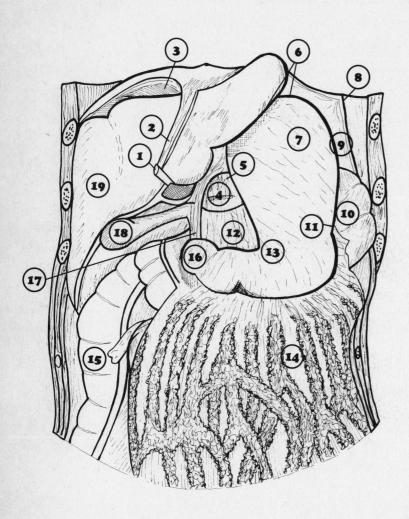

Lesser Omentum (Figs. 67A and 67B)

The visceral peritoneum covers the anterior surface of the stomach, and the lesser curvature forms the anterior layer of the lesser omentum. The lesser omentum has a free border on the right where it folds around the common bile duct, hepatic artery, and portal vein. This free border forms the anterior margin of the opening into the lesser sac. The peritoneum forms the posterior layer of the lesser omentum to become continuous with the visceral layer of peritoneum covering the posterior stomach wall.

The peritoneum leaves the greater curvature of the stomach to form the gastrosplenic omentum. At this point it reflects backward toward the abdominal wall to form the anterior layer of the lienorenal ligament. The peritoneum now covers the anterior surface of the pancreas, the aorta, and the inferior vena cava.

The peritoneum passes anteriorly over the right kidney to the lateral abdominal wall to reach the anterior abdominal wall, where it forms a continuous layer around the abdomen.

¹Ligamentum teres
²Falciform ligament
³Hepatic coronary ligament
⁴Caudate lobe of the liver
⁵Hepatogastric ligament
⁶Cardiac ligament
⁷Fundus of the stomach
⁸Diaphragm
⁹Parietal peritoneum
¹⁰Spleen
¹¹Gastrosplenic ligament
¹²Lesser omentum
¹³Lesser curvature of the stomach
¹⁴Greater omentum
¹⁵Ascending colon
¹⁶Pylorus
¹⁷Epiploic foramen
¹⁸Gallbladder
¹⁹Liver

Fig. 67B UPPER ABDOMEN (GREATER CURVATURE OF THE STOMACH LIFTED TO VIEW THE OMENTAL BURSA)

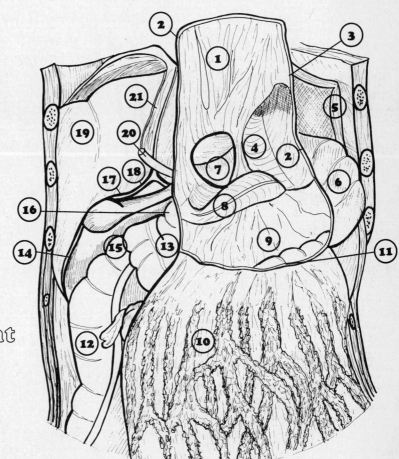

¹Stomach, pulled open
²Gastrosplenic ligament
³Phrenic gastric ligament
⁴Omental bursa
⁵Diaphragm
⁶Spleen
⁷Vestibule of the omental bursae
⁸Pancreas
⁹Transverse mesocolon
¹⁰Greater omentum
¹¹Gastrocolic ligament
¹²Ascending colon
¹³Transverse colon
¹⁴Anterior margin of the liver

¹⁵Hepatic flexure
¹⁶Pylorus
¹⁷Epiploic foramen
¹⁸Quadrate lobe of the liver
¹⁹Right lobe of the liver
²⁰Ligamentum teres
²¹Falciform ligament

Fig. 68 SAGITTAL SECTION THROUGH THE ABDOMEN AND PELVIS

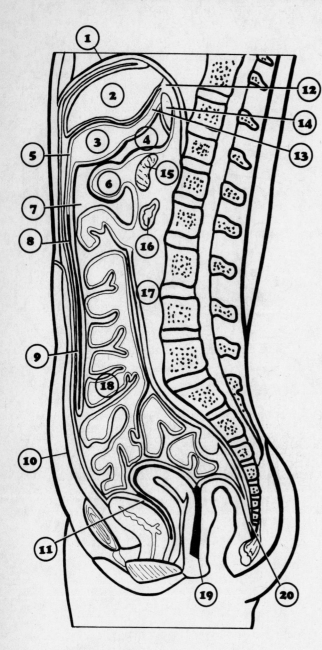

Sagittal View of the Peritoneum (Fig. 68)

The parietal peritoneum along the anterior abdominal wall may be traced from the falciform ligament to the diaphragm. The visceral peritoneum covers the anterior and inferior surfaces of the liver to the porta hepatis. At this point it passes to the lesser curvature of the stomach as the anterior layer of the lesser omentum. It covers the anterior surface of the stomach to form the greater omentum. The apron fold of the greater omentum hangs anterior to the intestine and contains part of the lesser sac within it. The peritoneum then folds upward and forms the posterior layer of the greater omentum. At the transverse colon the peritoneum forms the posterior layer of the transverse mesocolon. The peritoneum passes over the anterior border of the pancreas and runs downward anterior to the third part of the duodenum.

The peritoneum leaves the posterior abdominal wall as the anterior layer of the mesentery of the small intestine. The visceral peritoneum covers the jejunum and forms the posterior layer of the mesentery. The peritoneum returns to the posterior abdominal wall into the pelvis to cover the anterior rectum. Here, in the female, it reflects onto the posterior vagina to form the rectouterine pouch, or pouch of Douglas. In the female the peritoneum passes over the vagina to its anterior surface to the upper surface of the bladder to the anterior abdominal wall. In the male it reflects off the bladder and seminal vesicles to form the rectovesical pouch.

¹Diaphragm
²Liver
³Stomach
⁴Omental bursa
⁵Gastric ligament
⁶Transverse colon
⁷Peritoneal cavity
⁸Greater omentum
⁹Parietal peritoneum
¹⁰Linea alba
¹¹Vesicouterine pouch
¹²Subphrenic space
¹³Lesser omentum
¹⁴Caudate lobe of the liver
¹⁵Pancreas
¹⁶Duodenum
¹⁷Retroperitoneum
¹⁸Intestine
¹⁹Rectouterine pouch
²⁰Anococcygeus ligament

Gastrointestinal Tract
Fig. 69 PARTS OF THE DUODENUM

ESOPHAGUS AND STOMACH

The tubular esophagus descends from the thorax to enter the right side of the stomach through an opening in the right crus of the diaphragm. It is posterior to the left lobe of the liver and the left crus of the diaphragm.

The stomach lies under the ribs in the left upper abdomen. It extends from the left hypochrondriac region into the epigastric and umbilical regions. Its J-shaped structure has two openings (the cardiac and pyloric orifices), two curvatures (lesser and greater), and two surfaces (anterior and posterior).

It is usually divided into the following parts: fundus, body, pyloric antrum, and pyloris.

DUODENUM AND SMALL INTESTINE

Most of the digestion and absorption of food takes place in the small intestine. The small intestine is divided into three parts: the duodenum, the jejunum, and the ileum. The first section of the small intestine is the duodenum. The duodenum leads into the middle portion, the jejunum, and the small intestine then terminates in the ileum. The entire small intestine is about 23 feet long and 1 inch in diameter.

Duodenum

The duodenum is a C-shaped tube that curves around the head of the pancreas. The first few centimeters are covered with peritoneum, while the remainder lies retroperitoneally. The duodenum is generally divided into four parts for anatomical study (Fig. 69).

The first part (Fig. 70) begins at the pylorus and runs upward and backward on the right side of the first lumbar vertebra. It is related to the quadrate lobe of the liver and the gallbladder anteriorly; the lesser sac, the gastroduodenal artery, the common bile duct, the portal vein, and the inferior vena cava posteriorly; the epiploic foramen superiorly; and the head of the pancreas inferiorly.

The second part (Fig. 71) runs anterior to the left kidney on the right side of the second and third lumbar vertebrae. It is related to the fundus of the gallbladder, the right lobe of the liver, the transverse colon, and the small intestine anteriorly; the hilum of the right kidney posteriorly; the ascending colon, the right colic flexure, and the right lobe of the liver laterally; and the head of the pancreas medially. The common bile duct and main pancreatic duct pierce the duodenal wall midway down its posterior aspect.

The third part of the duodenum runs horizontally to the left, following the inferior margin of the pancreatic head. It is related to the root of the mesentery of the small intestine (and the superior mesenteric vessels) and the jejunum anteriorly; the right ureter, right psoas muscle, inferior vena cava, and aorta posteriorly; the head of the pancreas superiorly; and the jejunum inferiorly.

The fourth part of the duodenum runs upward and to the left, then runs forward at the duodenojejunal junction. (The ligament of Treitz ascends to the right crus and holds the junction in position.) It is related to the root of the mesentery and jejunum anteriorly and the left margin of the aorta and the medial border of the left psoas muscle posteriorly.

The upper half of the duodenum is supplied by the superior pancreaticoduodenal artery, and the lower half is supplied by the inferior pancreaticoduodenal artery. The veins of the duodenum drain into the portal circulation.

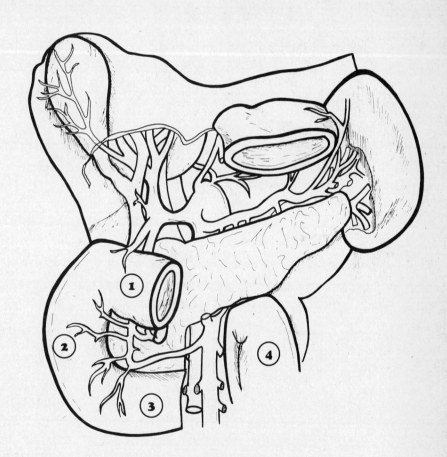

[1]First part of the duodenum (superior part)

[2]Second part of the duodenum (descending part)

[3]Third part of the duodenum (horizontal part)

[4]Fourth part of the duodenum

Fig. 70 ABDOMINAL SAGITTAL SECTION, LEVEL 5

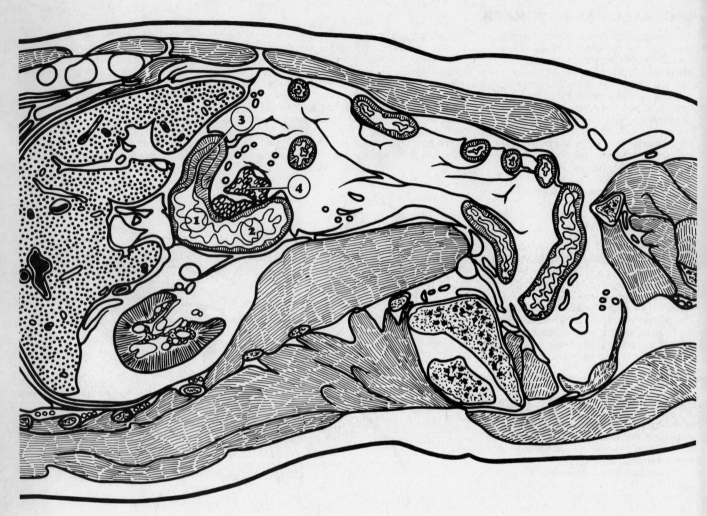

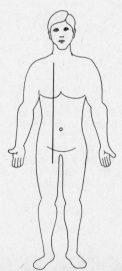

¹Superior duodenum
²Descending duodenum
³Pyloric sphincter
⁴Head of pancreas

Fig. 71 ABDOMINAL SAGITTAL SECTION, LEVEL 6

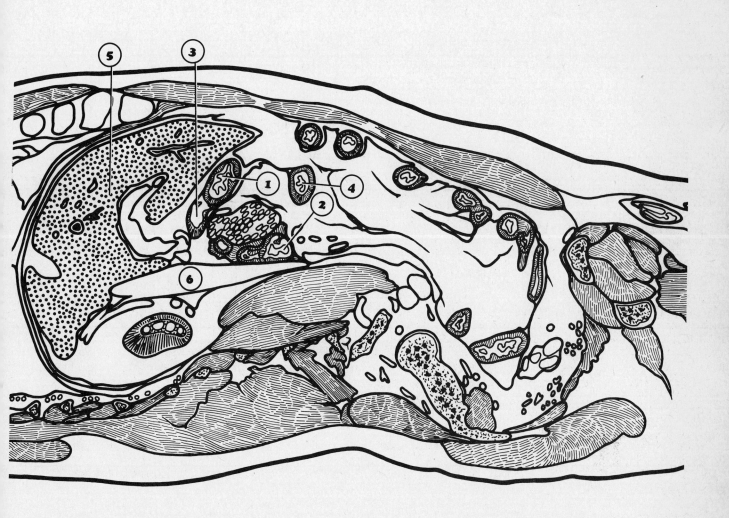

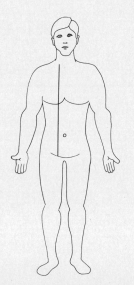

[1] Pyloric sphincter
[2] Superior part of the duodenum
[3] Descending part of the duodenum
[4] Transverse colon
[5] Right lobe of the liver
[6] Inferior vena cava

Liver

Fig. 72 ANTERIOR VIEW OF THE LIVER

The liver occupies almost all of the right hypochondrium, the greater part of the epigastrium, and usually the left hypochondrium to the mammillary line. It is divided into four regions: right lobe, left lobe, caudate lobe, and quadrate lobe.

LOBES OF THE LIVER

Right Lobe (Fig. 72)

The largest of the four lobes, the right lobe is six times larger than the left lobe. It occupies the right hypochondrium and is bordered on its upper surface by the falciform ligament, on its posterior surface by the left sagittal fossa, and on its anterior by the umbilical notch. The inferior and posterior surfaces are marked by the fossae of three structures: the porta hepatis, the gallbladder, and the inferior vena cava.

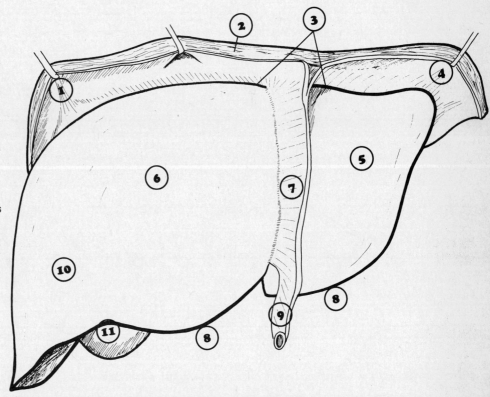

¹Right triangular ligament
²Diaphragm (pulled up)
³Coronary ligament
⁴Left triangular ligament
⁵Left lobe
⁶Right lobe
⁷Falciform ligament
⁸Inferior margin
⁹Ligamentum teres
¹⁰Costal impression
¹¹Gallbladder

Fig. 73 SUPERIOR VIEW OF THE LIVER

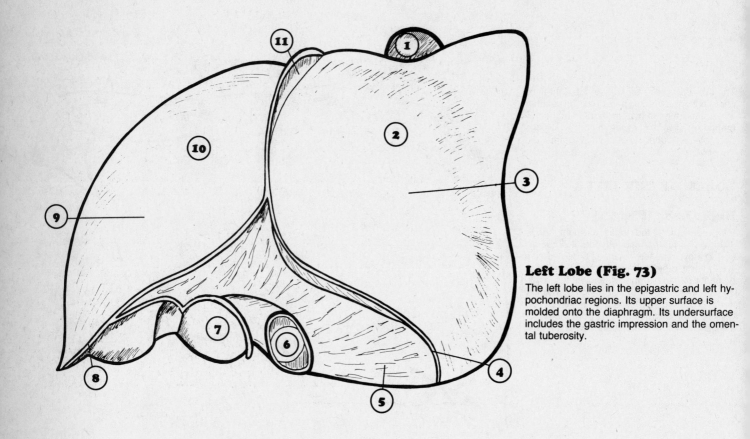

Left Lobe (Fig. 73)
The left lobe lies in the epigastric and left hypochondriac regions. Its upper surface is molded onto the diaphragm. Its undersurface includes the gastric impression and the omental tuberosity.

¹Fundus of the gallbladder
²Right lobe
³Diaphragmatic surface
⁴Coronary ligament
⁵Bare area
⁶Inferior vena cava
⁷Caudate lobe
⁸Left triangular ligament
⁹Diaphragmatic surface
¹⁰Left lobe
¹¹Falciform ligament

Fig. 74 POSTERIOR VIEW OF THE DIAPHRAGMATIC SURFACE OF THE LIVER

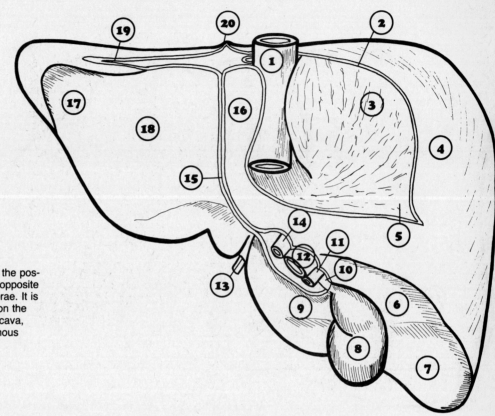

Caudate Lobe (Fig. 74)

The small, caudate lobe is located on the posterosuperior surface of the right lobe, opposite the tenth and eleventh thoracic vertebrae. It is bounded below by the porta hepatis, on the right by the fossa of the inferior vena cava, and on the left by the fossa of the venous duct.

[1] Inferior vena cava
[2] Coronary ligaments
[3] Bare area
[4] Right lobe
[5] Right triangular ligament
[6] Renal impression
[7] Colic impression
[8] Gallbladder
[9] Quadrate lobe
[10] Cystic duct
[11] Hepatic duct
[12] Portal vein
[13] Ligamentum teres
[14] Hepatic artery
[15] Attachment of the lesser omentum
[16] Caudate lobe
[17] Gastric impression
[18] Left lobe
[19] Left triangular ligament
[20] Falciform ligament

Fig. 75 INFERIOR VIEW OF THE VISCERAL SURFACE OF THE LIVER

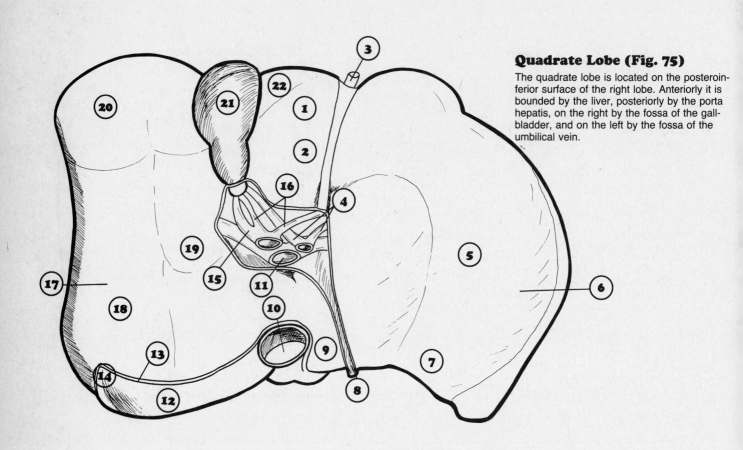

Quadrate Lobe (Fig. 75)

The quadrate lobe is located on the posteroinferior surface of the right lobe. Anteriorly it is bounded by the liver, posteriorly by the porta hepatis, on the right by the fossa of the gallbladder, and on the left by the fossa of the umbilical vein.

¹Quadrate lobe
²Pyloric area
³Ligamentum teres
⁴Hepatic arteries
⁵Gastric impression
⁶Left lobe
⁷Esophageal impression
⁸Ligamentum venosum
⁹Caudate lobe
¹⁰Inferior vena cava
¹¹Portal vein
¹²Bare area
¹³Coronary ligaments
¹⁴Right triangular ligament
¹⁵Cystic duct
¹⁶Hepatic ducts
¹⁷Right lobe
¹⁸Renal impression
¹⁹Duodenal impression
²⁰Colic impression
²¹Gallbladder
²²Colic impression

Fig. 76 VASCULAR SYSTEM OF THE LIVER

PORTAL AND HEPATIC VENOUS ANATOMY (Fig. 76)

The portal veins carry blood from the bowel to the liver; the hepatic veins drain the blood from the liver into the inferior vena cava. The hepatic arteries carry oxygenated blood from the aorta to the liver. The bile ducts transport bile, manufactured in the liver, to the duodenum.

Main Portal Vein

The main portal vein approaches the porta hepatis in a rightward, cephalad, and slightly posterior direction within the hepatoduodenal ligament. It comes into contact with the anterior surface of the inferior vena cava near the porta hepatis and serves to locate the liver hilum, where it divides into right and left portal veins.

Right Portal Vein

The right portal vein is the larger branch and requires a more posterior and caudal approach. The anterior division closely parallels the anterior abdominal wall.

Left Portal Vein

The left portal vein is more anterior and cranial than is the right portal vein. The main portal vein elongates at the origin of the left portal vein.

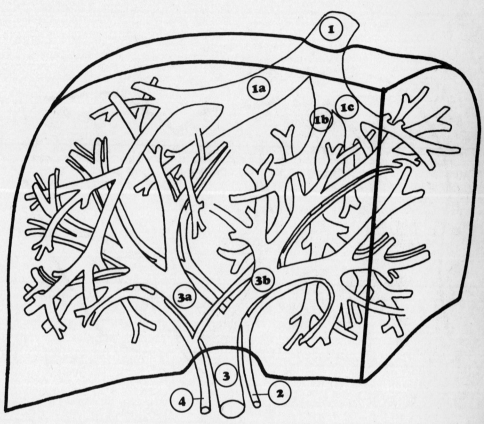

¹Hepatic veins
¹ᵃRight hepatic
¹ᵇMiddle hepatic
¹ᶜLeft hepatic
²Hepatic artery
³Portal vein
³ᵃRight portal
³ᵇLeft portal
⁴Bile duct

Fig. 77 HEPATIC VEINS

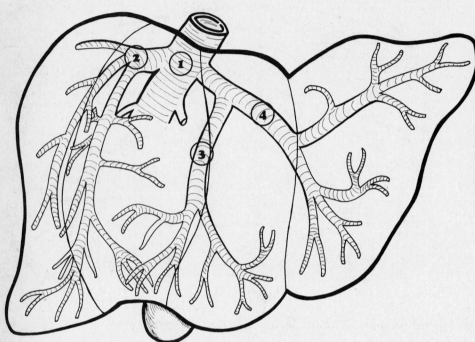

Hepatic Veins (Fig. 77)

The hepatic veins are divided into three components: right, middle, and left. The right hepatic vein is the largest and enters the right lateral aspect of the inferior vena cava. The middle hepatic vein enters the anterior or right anterior surface of the inferior vena cava. The left hepatic vein enters the left anterior surface of the inferior vena cava.

¹Inferior vena cava
²Right hepatic vein
³Middle hepatic vein
⁴Left hepatic vein

Fig. 78 DIVISIONS OF THE LIVER

SEGMENTAL LIVER ANATOMY

The liver is divided into two lobes, right and left, each of which has two segments (Fig. 78). The right lobe is divided into anterior and posterior segments, the left lobe into medial and lateral segments. The quadrate lobe is a portion of the medial segment. The caudate lobe is the posterior portion of the liver lying between the fossa of the inferior vena cava and the fissure of the ligamentum venosum. The caudate lobe receives portal venous and hepatic arterial blood from both the right and left systems.

Functional Division of the Liver

The purpose of a functional division is to separate the liver into component parts according to blood supply and biliary drainage so that one component can be removed in the event of tumor invasion or trauma.

The right functional lobe includes everything to the right of a plane through the gallbladder fossa and inferior vena cava. The left functional lobe includes everything to the left of this plane.

LIGAMENTS AND FISSURES

There are several important ligaments and fissures in the liver. The falciform ligament extends from the umbilicus to the diaphragm in a parasagittal plane. Within this ligament is a round fibrous cord, the ligamentum teres, a remnant of the old umbilical vein. In the anteroposterior axis the falciform ligament extends from the right rectus muscle to the bare area of the liver.

The bare area of the liver is where the peritoneal reflections from the liver onto the diaphragm leave an irregular triangle of liver without peritoneal covering. The peritoneal reflections around the bare area are called the coronary ligament. The caudal part of the coronary ligament is reflected onto the diaphragm and the right kidney and is called the hepatorenal ligament. Below this is a potential peritoneal space, the hepatorenal pouch, (pouch of Morison), which is bounded by the liver, kidney, colon, and duodenum.

Both the falciform ligament and the ligamentum teres divide the medial segments of the left lobe. The fissure for the ligamentum venosum separates the left lobe from the caudate lobe.

RELATIONAL ANATOMY

The fundus of the stomach lies posterior and lateral to the left lobe of the liver. The duodenum lies adjacent to the right and quadrate lobes of the liver. The pancreas is usually just inferior to the liver. The posterior border impinges on the right kidney, inferior vena cava, and aorta. The diaphragm covers the superior border of the liver.

SUBPHRENIC SPACES

The right and left anterior subphrenic spaces lie between the diaphragm and the liver on each side of the falciform ligament. The right posterior subphrenic space lies amid the right lobe of the liver, the right kidney, and the right colic flexure. The right extraperitoneal space lies between the layers of the coronary ligament between the liver and diaphragm.

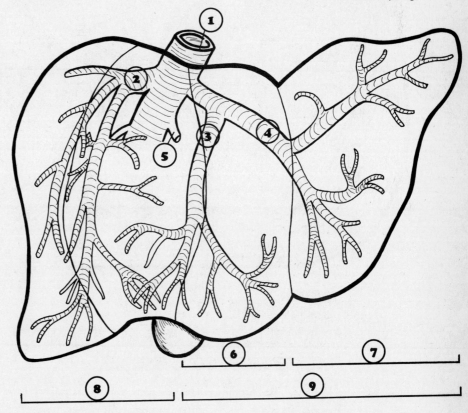

¹Inferior vena cava
²Right hepatic vein
³Middle hepatic vein
⁴Left hepatic vein
⁵Caudate lobe

⁶Medial segment
⁷Lateral segment
⁸Right lobe
⁹Left lobe

Fig. 79 SERIAL CROSS SECTION OF THE LIVER, LEVEL 1

SERIAL CROSS SECTIONS OF THE LIVER (Figs. 79 Through 85)

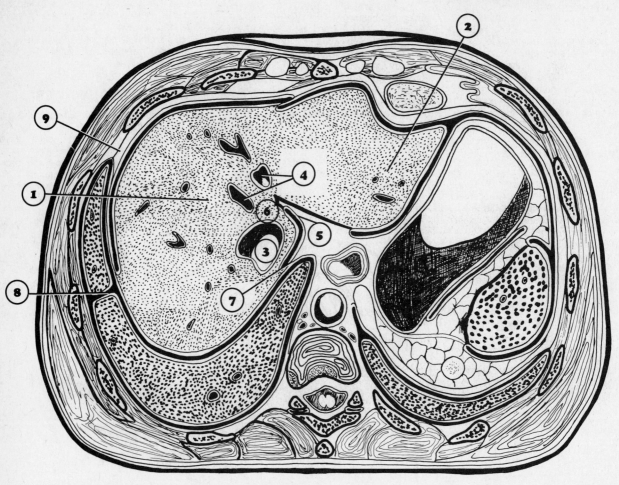

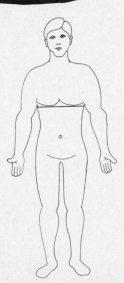

¹Right lobe
²Left lobe
³Inferior vena cava
⁴Hepatic vein
⁵Ligamentum venosum
⁶Caudate lobe
⁷Coronary hepatic ligament
⁸Pleural cavity
⁹Diaphragm

Fig. 80 SERIAL CROSS SECTION OF THE LIVER, LEVEL 2

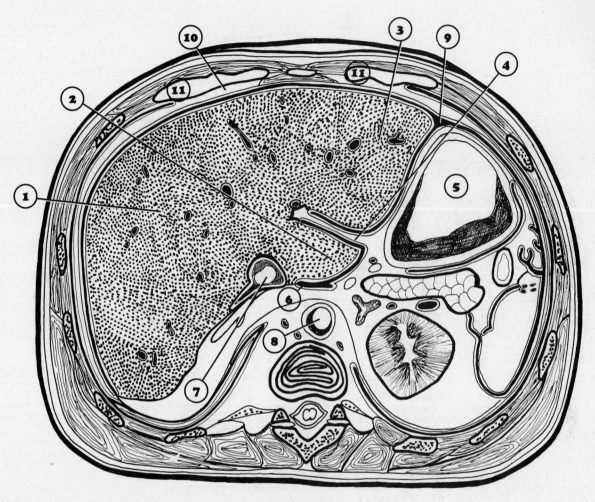

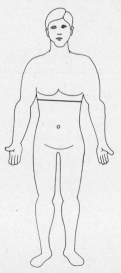

1 Right lobe
2 Caudate lobe
3 Left lobe
4 Hepatogastric ligament
5 Stomach
6 Omental bursa
7 Inferior vena cava
8 Aorta
9 Peritoneal cavity
10 Diaphragm
11 Rectus abdominis
   muscle

Fig. 81 SERIAL CROSS SECTION OF THE LIVER, LEVEL 3

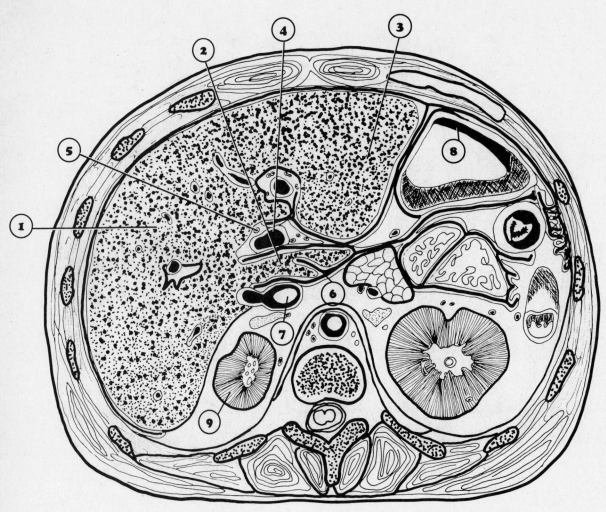

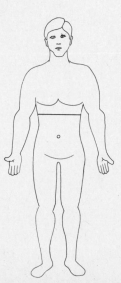

¹Right lobe
²Caudate lobe
³Left lobe
⁴Portal vein
⁵Hepatic duct
⁶Omental bursa
⁷Inferior vena cava
⁸Stomach
⁹Right kidney

Fig. 82 SERIAL CROSS SECTION OF THE LIVER, LEVEL 4

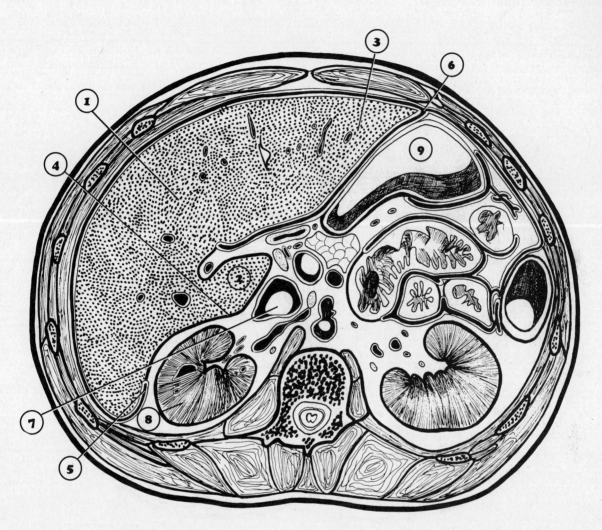

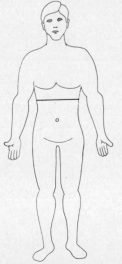

[1]Right lobe
[2]Caudate lobe
[3]Left lobe
[4]Epiploic foramen
[5]Hepatorenal ligament
[6]Peritoneum
[7]Inferior vena cava
[8]Right kidney
[9]Stomach

Fig. 83 SERIAL CROSS SECTION OF THE LIVER, LEVEL 5

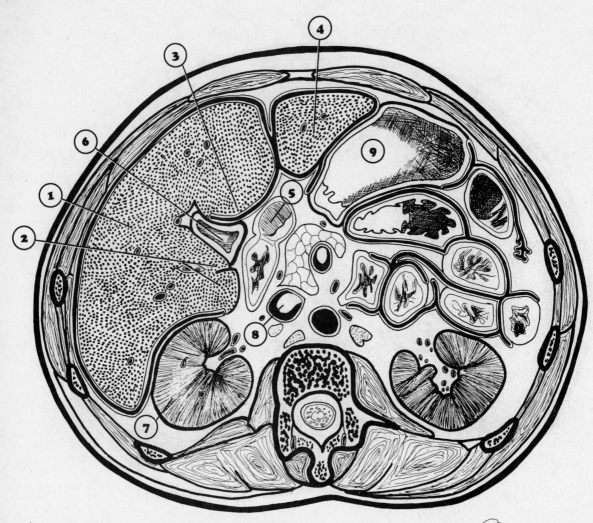

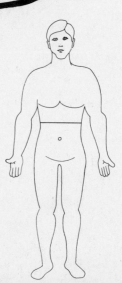

[1]Right lobe
[2]Caudate lobe
[3]Quadrate lobe
[4]Left lobe
[5]Duodenum
[6]Gallbladder
[7]Right kidney
[8]Inferior vena cava
[9]Stomach

Fig. 84 SERIAL CROSS SECTION OF THE LIVER, LEVEL 6

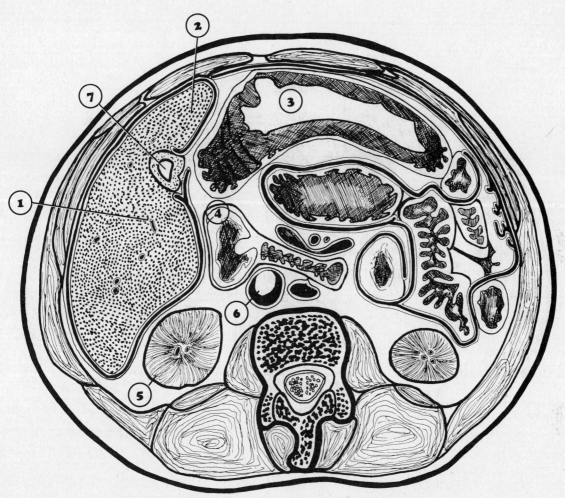

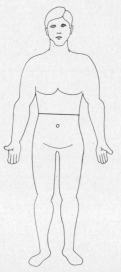

¹Right lobe
²Quadrate lobe
³Stomach
⁴Duodenum
⁵Right kidney
⁶Inferior vena cava
⁷Gallbladder

Fig. 85 SERIAL CROSS SECTION OF THE LIVER, LEVEL 7

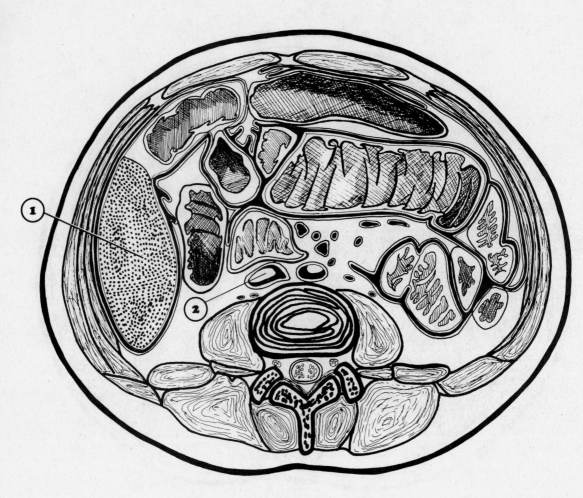

¹Right lobe
²Inferior vena cava

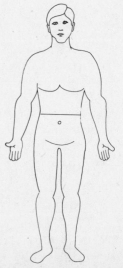

Fig. 86 ABDOMINAL SAGITTAL SECTION, LEVEL 1

**SERIAL SAGITTAL
SECTIONS OF THE LIVER
(Figs. 86 Through 96)**

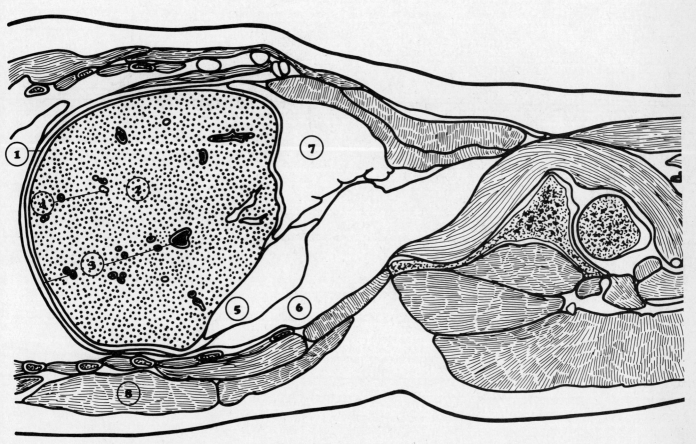

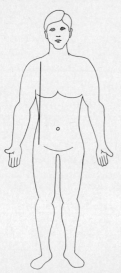

¹Diaphragm
²Right lobe
³Hepatic vein
⁴Portal vein
⁵Perirenal fat
⁶Retroperitoneal fat
⁷Omentum
⁸Latissimus dorsi muscle

Fig. 87 ABDOMINAL SAGITTAL SECTION, LEVEL 2

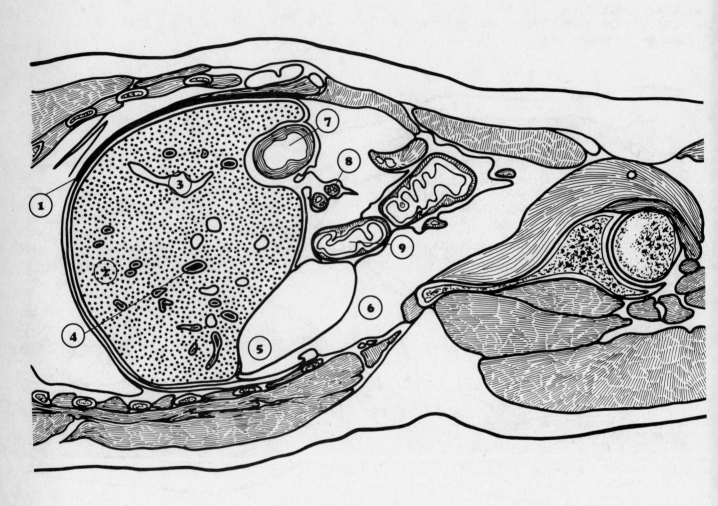

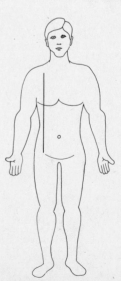

[1] Diaphragm
[2] Right lobe
[3] Portal vein
[4] Hepatic vein
[5] Perirenal fat
[6] Retroperitoneal fat
[7] Gallbladder
[8] Hepatic flexure
[9] Ascending colon

Fig. 88 ABDOMINAL SAGITTAL SECTION, LEVEL 3

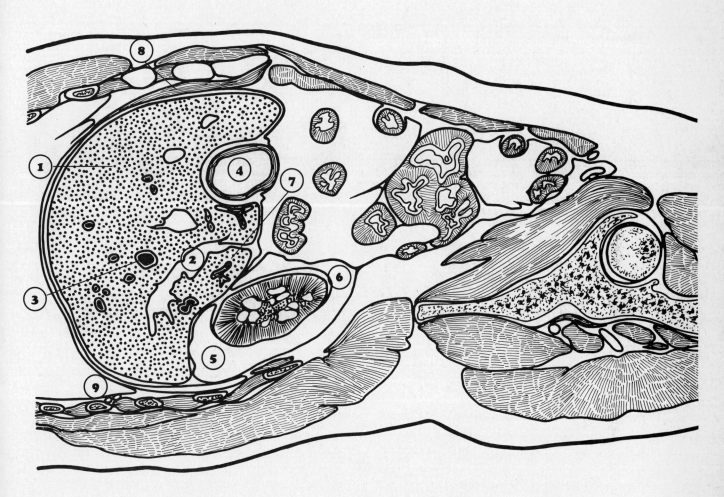

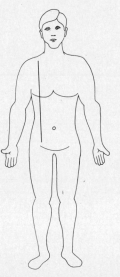

¹Right lobe
²Portal vein
³Hepatic vein
⁴Gallbladder
⁵Right kidney
⁶Perirenal fat
⁷Caudate lobe
⁸Diaphragm
⁹Costodiaphragmatic recess

Fig. 89 ABDOMINAL SAGITTAL SECTION, LEVEL 4

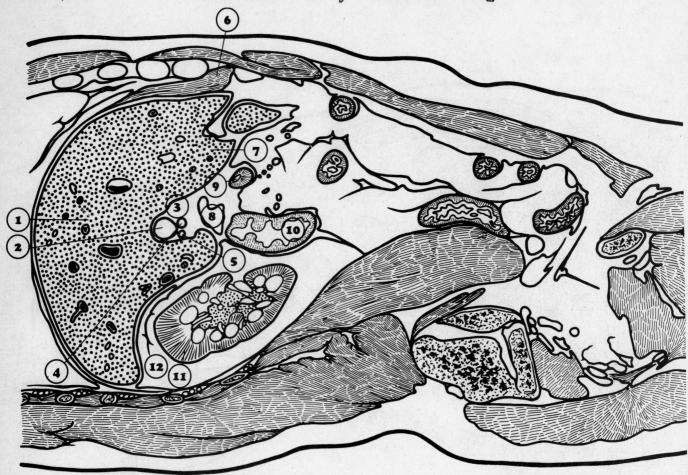

¹Right lobe
²Right portal vein
³Porta hepatis
⁴Hepatic artery
⁵Common bile duct
⁶Diaphragm
⁷Quadrate lobe
⁸Neck of gallbladder
⁹Superior part of the
  duodenum
¹⁰Descending part of the
  duodenum
¹¹Right kidney
¹²Perirenal fat

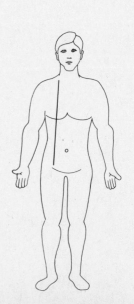

Fig. 90 ABDOMINAL SAGITTAL SECTION, LEVEL 5

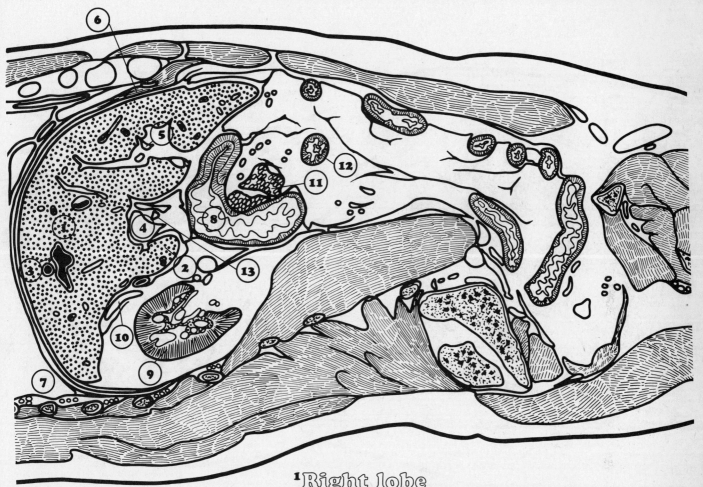

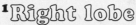

[1]Right lobe
[2]Caudate lobe
[3]Hepatic vein
[4]Portal vein
[5]Left portal vein
[6]Diaphragm
[7]Costodiaphragmatic
    recess
[8]Duodenum
[9]Right kidney
[10]Right suprarenal gland
[11]Pancreas
[12]Transverse colon
[13]Cystic duct

Fig. 91 ABDOMINAL SAGITTAL SECTION, LEVEL 6

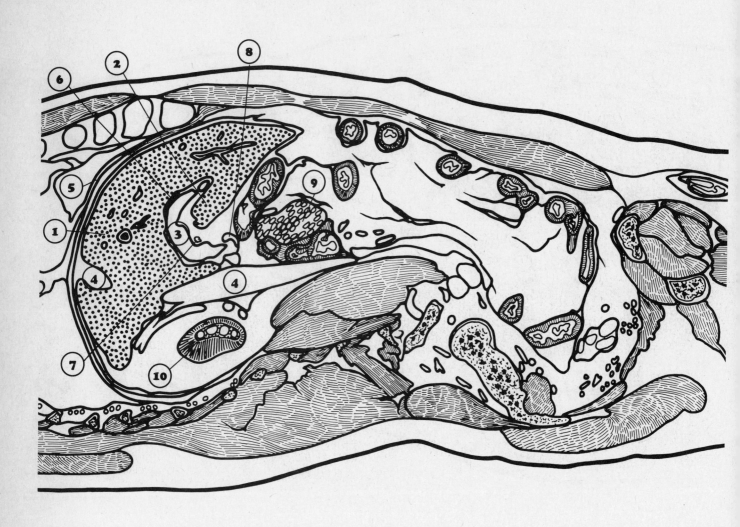

1 Right lobe
2 Caudate lobe
3 Left portal vein
4 Inferior vena cava
5 Diaphragm
6 Fissure for the
   ligamentum teres
7 Hepatic artery
8 Common bile duct
9 Head of the pancreas
10 Right kidney

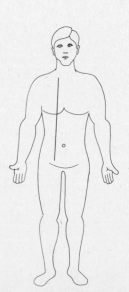

Fig. 92 ABDOMINAL SAGITTAL SECTION, LEVEL 7

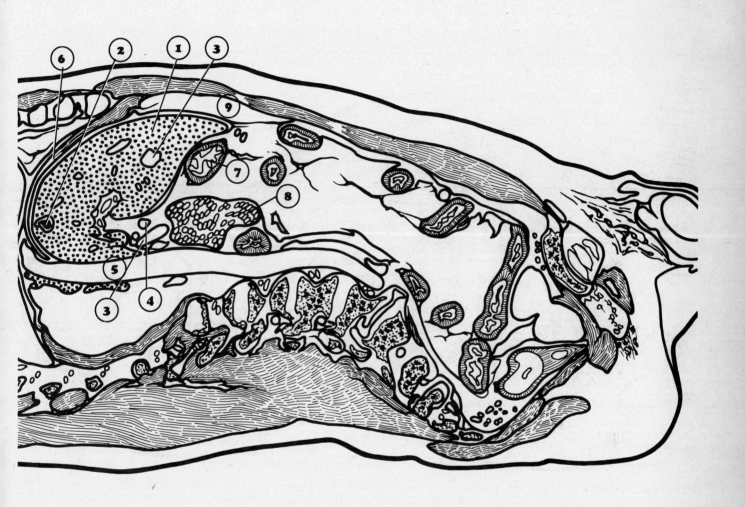

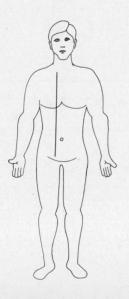

1 Left lobe
2 Hepatic vein
3 Portal vein
4 Hepatic artery
5 Inferior vena cava
6 Diaphragm
7 Pyloric antrum
8 Pancreas
9 Falciform ligament

Fig. 93 ABDOMINAL SAGITTAL SECTION, LEVEL 8

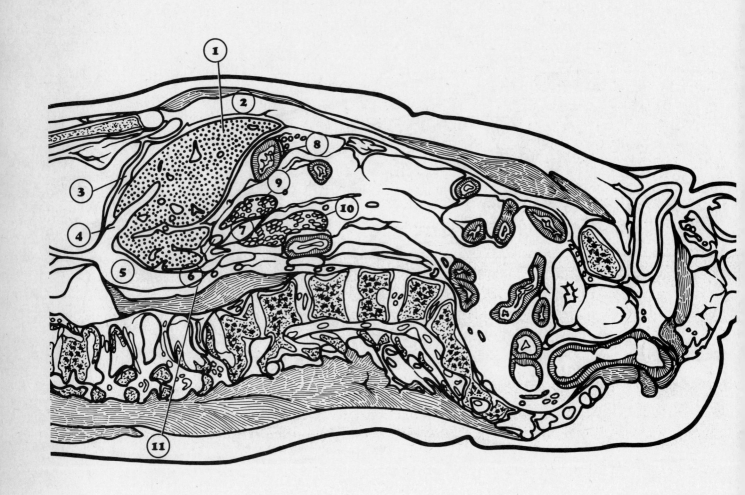

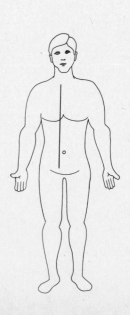

¹Left lobe
²Falciform ligament
³Diaphragm
⁴Hepatic vein
⁵Inferior vena cava
⁶Hepatic artery
⁷Portal vein
⁸Pyloric antrum
⁹Pancreatic head
¹⁰Uncinate process
¹¹Crus of the diaphragm

Fig. 94 ABDOMINAL SAGITTAL SECTION, LEVEL 9

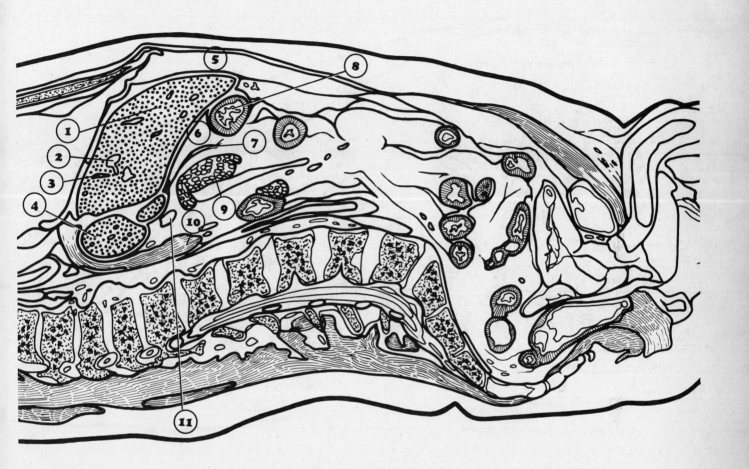

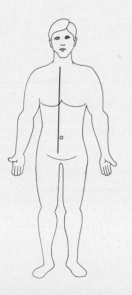

1 Left lobe
2 Portal vein
3 Hepatic vein
4 Caudate lobe
5 Falciform ligament
6 Lesser omentum
7 Lesser sac
8 Pyloric antrum
9 Pancreas
10 Crus of the diaphragm
11 Hepatic artery

Fig. 95 ABDOMINAL SAGITTAL SECTION, LEVEL 10

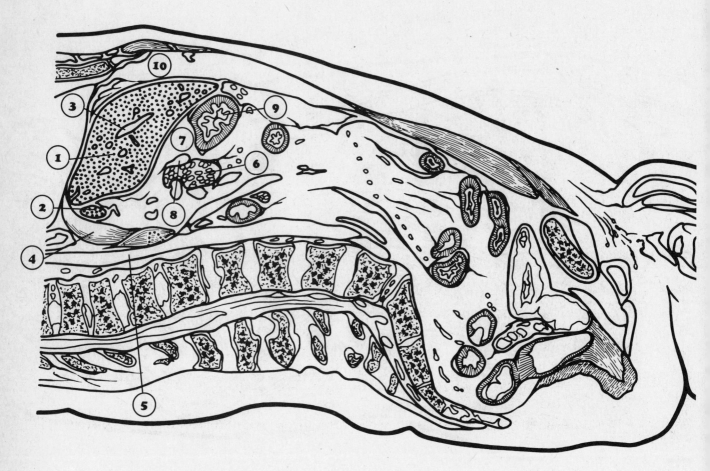

1 Left lobe
2 Caudate lobe
3 Portal vein
4 Crus of the diaphragm
5 Aorta
6 Pancreas
7 Lesser omentum
8 Lesser sac
9 Stomach
10 Falciform ligament

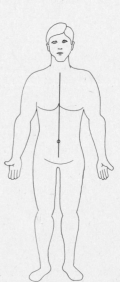

Fig. 96 ABDOMINAL SAGITTAL SECTION, LEVEL 11

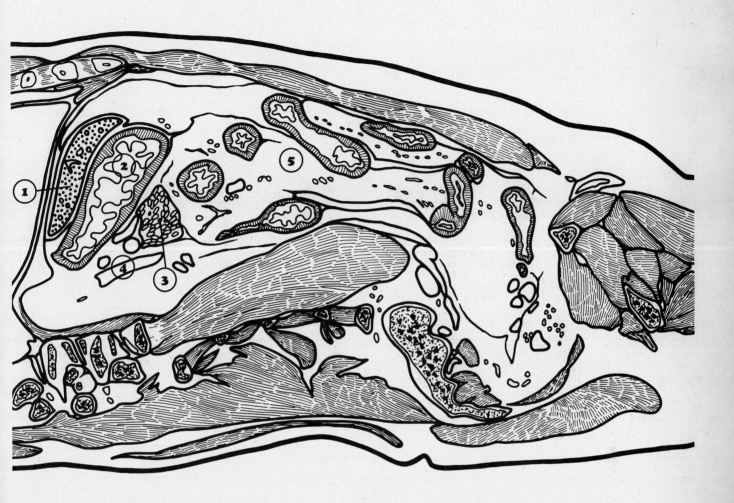

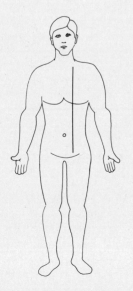

[1]Left lobe
[2]Body of stomach
[3]Pancreas
[4]Left suprarenal gland
[5]Mesentery

Gallbladder and Biliary System

Fig. 97 ANTERIOR VIEW OF THE BILIARY SYSTEM

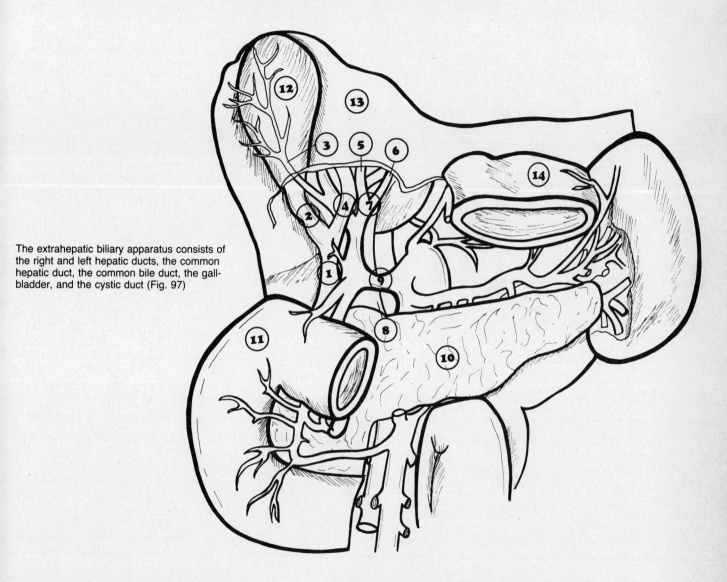

The extrahepatic biliary apparatus consists of the right and left hepatic ducts, the common hepatic duct, the common bile duct, the gall-bladder, and the cystic duct (Fig. 97)

¹Common bile duct
²Cystic duct
³Cystic artery
⁴Common hepatic duct
⁵Middle hepatic artery
⁶Left hepatic artery
⁷Proper hepatic artery
⁸Portal vein
⁹Common hepatic artery
¹⁰Pancreas
¹¹Duodenum
¹²Gallbladder
¹³Liver
¹⁴Stomach

Fig. 98 GALLBLADDER AND BILE DUCTS

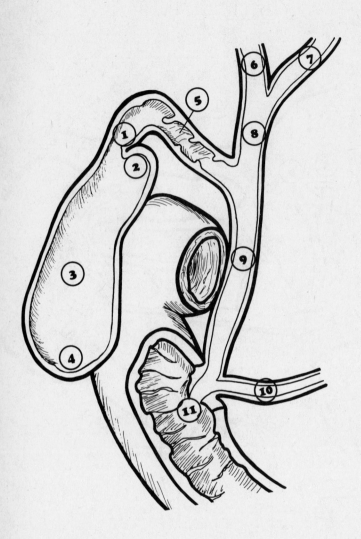

HEPATIC DUCTS (FIG. 98)

The right and left hepatic ducts emerge from the right lobe of the liver in the porta hepatis to form the common hepatic duct. The hepatic duct passes caudally and medially and runs parallel to the portal vein.

The common hepatic duct is approximately 4 mm in diameter and descends into the edge of the lesser omentum. It is joined by the cystic duct to form the common bile duct.

¹Neck of gallbladder
²Hartmann's pouch
³Body of the gallbladder
⁴Fundus of the gallbladder
⁵Cystic duct
⁶Right hepatic duct
⁷Left hepatic duct
⁸Common hepatic duct
⁹Common bile duct
¹⁰Pancreatic duct
¹¹Papilla of Vater

Fig. 99 GALLBLADDER AND BILE DUCTS

COMMON BILE DUCT (Fig. 99)

The common bile duct has a diameter of less than 6 mm. In the first part of its course it lies in the right free edge of the lesser omentum. In the second part it is situated posterior to the first part of the duodenum. In the third part it lies in a groove on the posterior surface of the head of the pancreas. It ends by piercing the medial wall of the second part of the duodenum. There, it is joined by the main pancreatic duct, and together, they open through the small ampulla of Vater into the duodenal wall. The ends of both ducts and the ampulla are surrounded by circular muscle fibers known as the sphincter of Oddi.

The proximal portion of the common bile duct is lateral to the hepatic artery and anterior to the portal vein. The duct becomes more posterior after it descends behind the duodenal bulb and enters the pancreas. The distal duct lies parallel to the anterior wall of the vena cava.

Within the liver parenchyma, the bile ducts follow the same course as the portal venous and hepatic arterial branches. All of the structures are encased in a common collagenous sheath forming the portal triad.

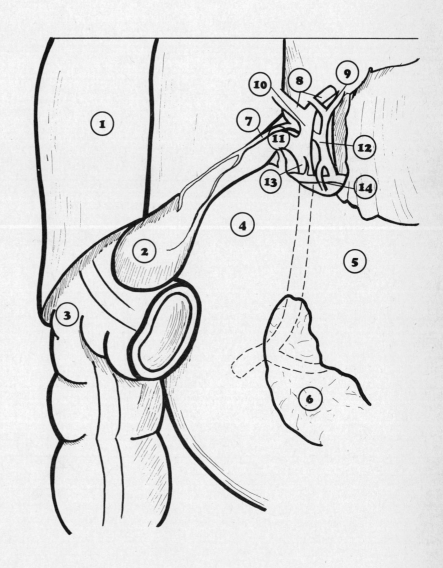

¹Liver
²Gallbladder
³Colon
⁴Duodenum
⁵Stomach
⁶Pancreas
⁷Cystic artery
⁸Right and left hepatic ducts
⁹Right and left hepatic arteries
¹⁰Common hepatic duct
¹¹Cystic duct
¹²Proper hepatic artery
¹³Common bile duct
¹⁴Right gastric artery

Fig. 100 POSTERIOR VIEW OF THE DIAPHRAGMATIC SURFACE OF THE GALLBLADDER

GALLBLADDER

The gallbladder is a pear-shaped sac in the anterior aspect of the right upper quadrant, closely related to the visceral surface of the liver (Figs. 100 and 101). It is divided into the fundus, body, and neck. The fundus usually projects below the inferior margin of the liver, where it comes into contact with the anterior abdominal wall at the level of the ninth right costal cartilage. The body generally lies in contact with the visceral surface of the liver and is directed upward, backward, and to the left (Fig. 102). The neck becomes continuous with the cystic duct, which turns into the lesser omentum to join the right side of the common hepatic duct to form the common bile duct (Fig. 103).

The neck of the gallbladder is oriented posteromedially toward the porta hepatis; the fundus is lateral, caudal, and anterior to the neck.

The arterial supply of the gallbladder is from the cystic artery, a branch of the right hepatic artery. The cystic vein drains directly into the portal vein. A number of smaller arteries and veins run between the liver and the gallbladder.

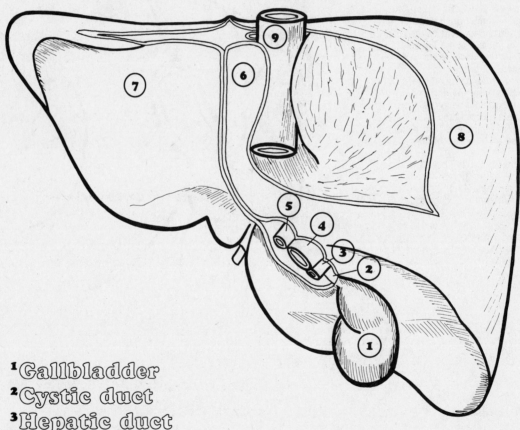

¹Gallbladder
²Cystic duct
³Hepatic duct
⁴Portal vein
⁵Hepatic artery
⁶Caudate lobe of the liver
⁷Left lobe of the liver
⁸Right lobe of the liver
⁹Inferior vena cava

Fig. 101 INFERIOR VIEW OF THE VISCERAL SURFACE OF THE GALLBLADDER

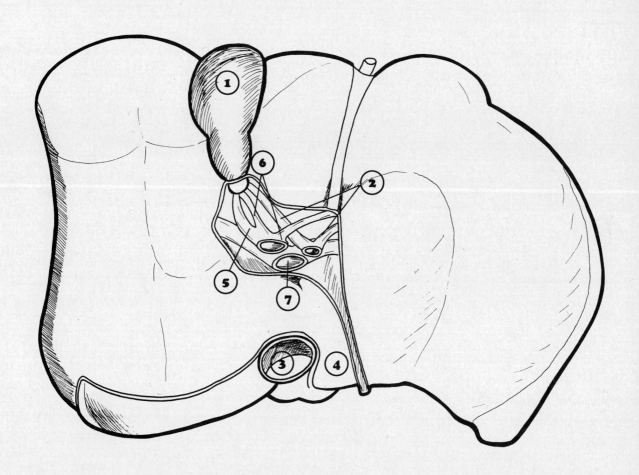

¹Gallbladder
²Hepatic arteries
³Inferior vena cava
⁴Caudate lobe of the
    liver
⁵Cystic duct
⁶Hepatic ducts
⁷Portal vein

Fig. 102 GALLBLADDER AND SURROUNDING ORGANS

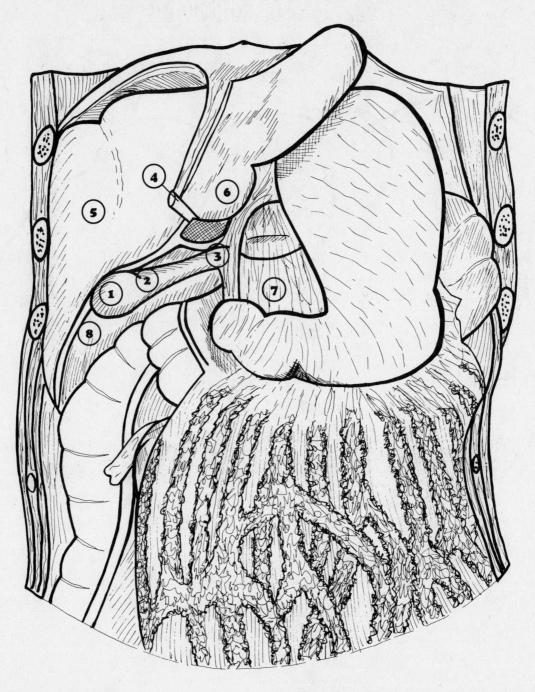

¹Fundus of the gallbladder
²Body of the gallbladder
³Neck of the gallbladder
⁴Ligamentum teres
⁵Right lobe of the liver
⁶Caudate lobe of the liver
⁷Lesser sac
⁸Duodenum

Fig. 103 ANTERIOR CORONAL VIEW OF THE GALLBLADDER

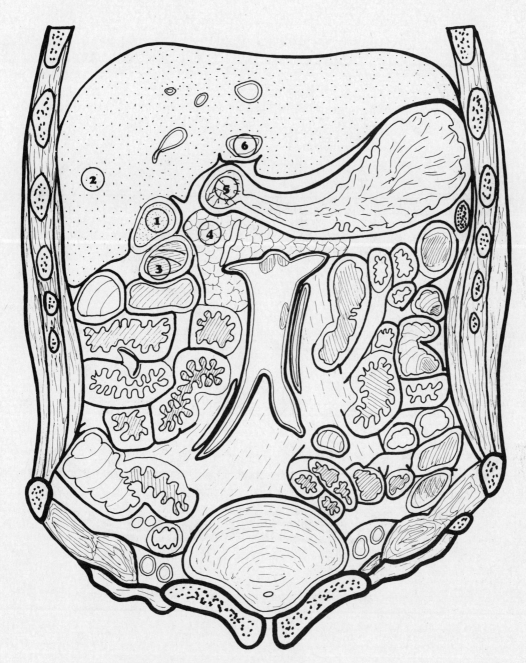

[1] Gallbladder
[2] Right lobe of the liver
[3] Transverse colon
[4] Head of the pancreas
[5] Duodenum
[6] Portal vein

Fig. 104 SERIAL CROSS SECTION OF THE GALLBLADDER, LEVEL 5

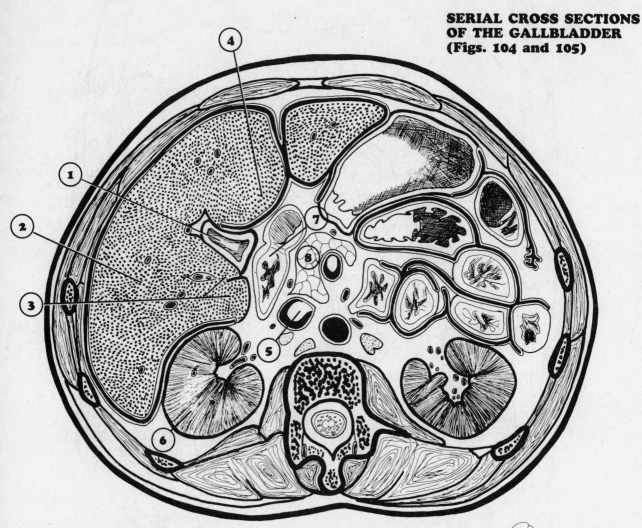

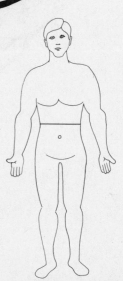

¹Gallbladder
²Right lobe of the liver
³Caudate lobe of the liver
⁴Quadrate lobe of the liver
⁵Inferior vena cava
⁶Right kidney
⁷Duodenum
⁸Pancreas

Fig. 105 SERIAL CROSS SECTION OF THE GALLBLADDER, LEVEL 6

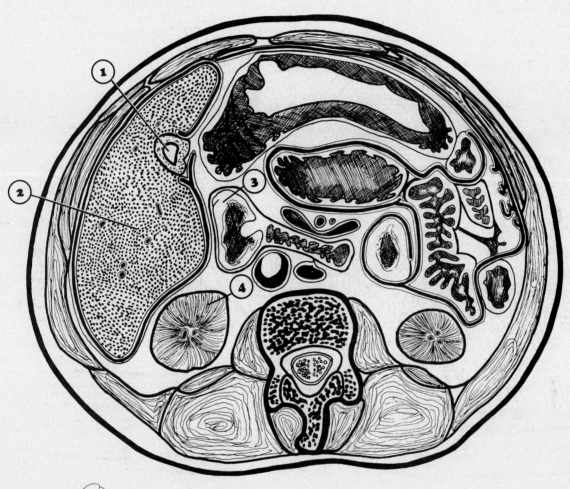

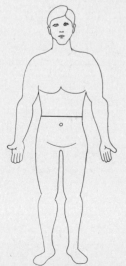

[1]Gallbladder
[2]Right lobe of the liver
[3]Duodenum
[4]Right kidney

Fig. 106 ABDOMINAL SAGITTAL SECTION, LEVEL 2

SERIAL SAGITTAL SECTIONS OF THE GALLBLADDER (Figs. 106 Through 108)

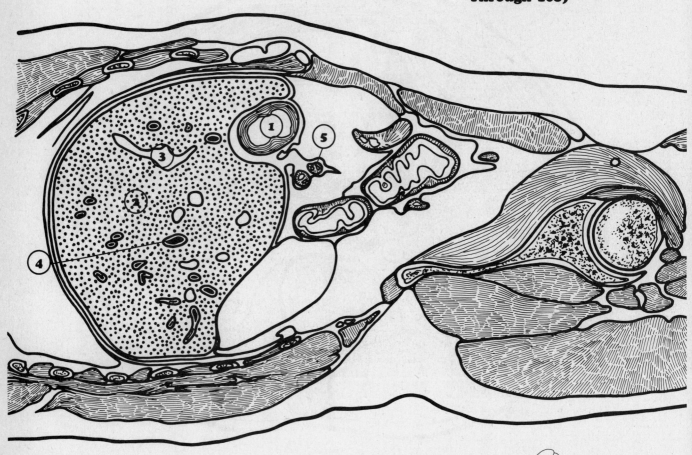

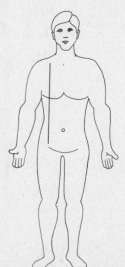

¹Gallbladder
²Right lobe of the liver
³Portal vein
⁴Hepatic vein
⁵Hepatic flexure

Fig. 107 ABDOMINAL SAGITTAL SECTION, LEVEL 3

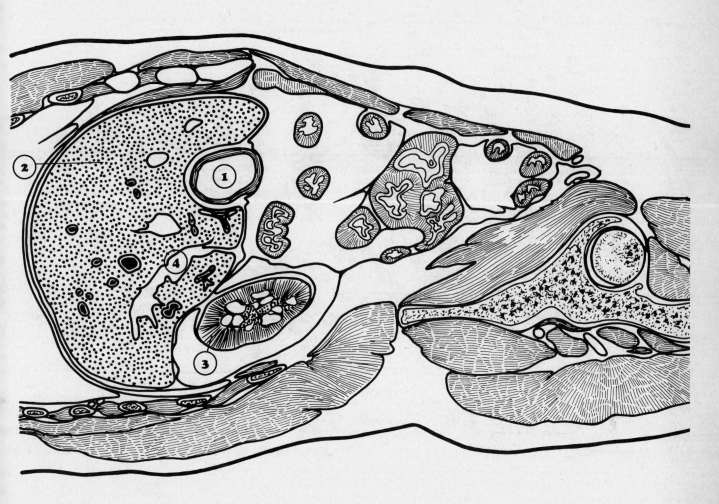

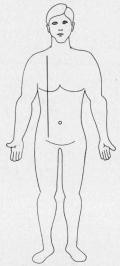

¹Gallbladder
²Right lobe of the liver
³Right kidney
⁴Portal vein

113

Fig. 108 ABDOMINAL SAGITTAL SECTION, LEVEL 4

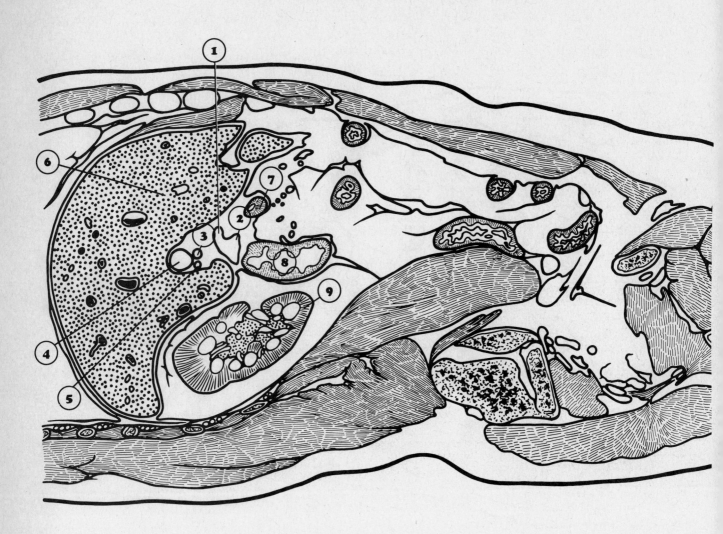

1 Neck of gallbladder
2 Hartmann's pouch
3 Common bile duct
4 Hepatic artery
5 Right portal vein
6 Right lobe of the liver
7 Superior part of the duodenum
8 Descending part of the duodenum
9 Right kidney

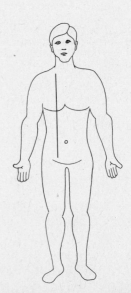

Vascular Structures

Fig. 109 CROSS SECTION OF A VEIN AND AN ARTERY

GENERAL COMPOSITION OF VESSELS

Blood is carried away from the heart by the arteries and is returned from the tissues to the heart by the veins. Arteries divide into smaller and smaller branches, the smallest of which are the arterioles. These lead into the capillaries, which are minute vessels that branch and form a network where the exchange of materials between blood and tissue fluid takes place. After the blood passes through the capillaries, it is collected into the small veins, or venules. These small vessels unite to form larger vessels that eventually return the blood to the heart for recirculation.

A typical artery in cross section consists of three layers (Fig. 109):

The tunica intima (inner layer), which itself consists of three layers:
   A layer of endothelial cells that line the arterial passage (lumen)
   A layer of delicate connective tissue
   An elastic layer made up of a network of elastic fibers

The tunica media (middle layer), which consists of smooth muscle fibers with elastic and collagenous tissue

The tunica adventitia (external layer), which is composed of loose connective tissue with bundles of smooth muscle fibers and elastic tissue

Smaller arteries contain less elastic tissue and more smooth muscle. The elasticity of the large arteries is vital to the maintenance of a steady blood flow.

The veins have the same three layers as do the arteries, but they differ in that their tunica media is thinner. They appear collapsed owing to the little elastic tissue or muscle in their walls.

Veins have special valves within them that permit blood to flow only in one direction, toward the heart. They have a larger total diameter than do arteries, and the blood moves toward the heart slowly, as compared with the arterial circulation.

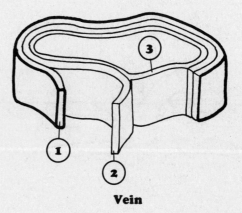

Vein

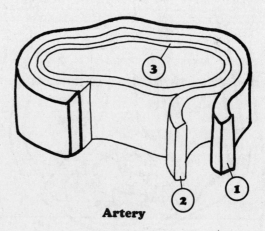

Artery

[1]Tunica adventitia
[2]Tunica media
[3]Tunica intima

Fig. 110

INFERIOR VENA CAVA AND ITS TRIBUTARIES

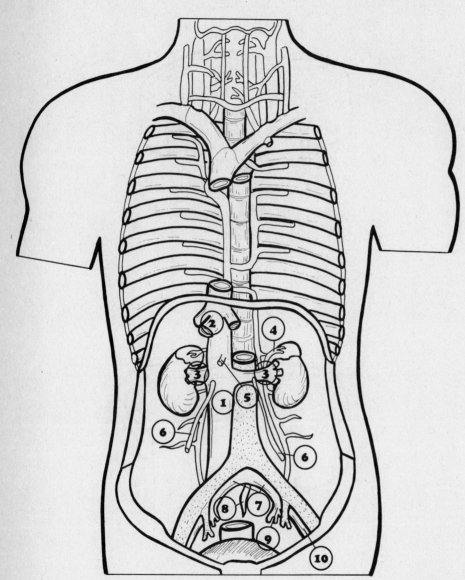

MAIN SYSTEM VEINS

Inferior Vena Cava (Figs. 110 and 111)

The inferior vena cava is formed by the union of the common iliac veins behind the right common iliac artery. It ascends vertically through the retroperitoneal space on the right side of the aorta posterior to the liver, piercing the central tendon of the diaphragm at the level of the eighth thoracic vertebrae and enters the right atrium of the heart. Its entrance into the lesser sac separates it from the portal vein.

The tributaries of the inferior vena cava are the hepatic veins, the right adrenal veins, the renal veins, the right testicular or ovarian vein, the inferior phrenic vein, the four lumbar veins, the common iliac veins, and the median sacral vein.

[1] Inferior vena cava
[2] Hepatic vein
[3] Renal veins
[4] Suprarenal vein
[5] Phrenic vein
[6] Testicular or ovarian veins
[7] Common iliac (right and left) veins
[8] Middle sacral vein
[9] Internal iliac vein
[10] External iliac vein

Fig. 111 AZYGOS VEIN AND ITS TRIBUTARIES

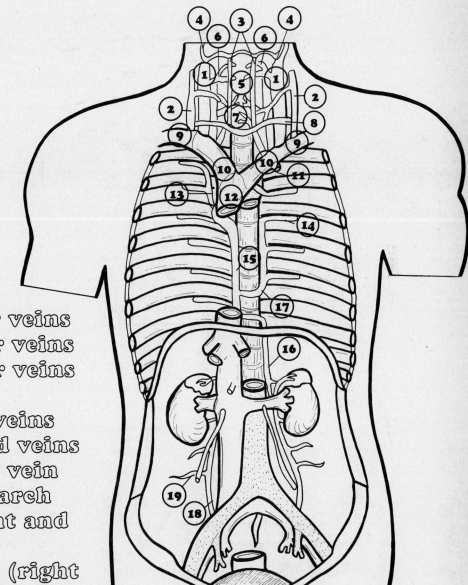

¹Internal jugular veins
²External jugular veins
³Anterior jugular veins
⁴Facial veins
⁵Middle thyroid veins
⁶Superior thyroid veins
⁷Inferior thyroid vein
⁸Jugular venous arch
⁹Subclavian (right and left) veins
¹⁰Brachiocephalic (right and left) veins
¹¹Internal thoracic vein
¹²Superior vena cava
¹³Superior intercostal vein
¹⁴Posterior intercostal vein
¹⁵Azygos vein

¹⁶Hemiazygos vein
¹⁷Accessory hemiazygos vein
¹⁸Ascending lumbar vein
¹⁹Lumbar vein

Fig. 112 PORTAL VENOUS SUPPLY IN THE LIVER

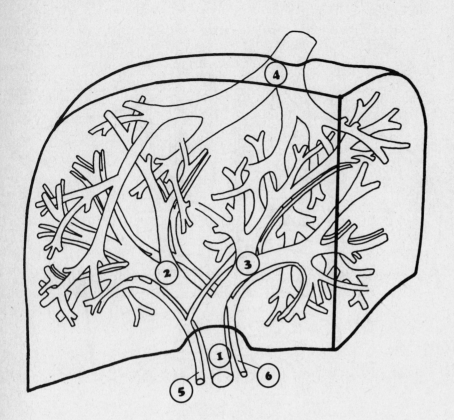

Portal Vein (Fig. 112)

The portal vein is formed posterior to the pancreas by the union of the superior mesenteric and splenic veins. It runs upward and to the right, posterior to the first part of the duodenum, and enters the lesser omentum. It then ascends anterior to the opening into the lesser sac to the porta hepatis, where it divides into right and left terminal branches. It drains blood out of the gastrointestinal tract from the lower end of the esophagus to the upper end of the anal canal, from the pancreas, gallbladder, and bile ducts, and from the spleen. It has an important anastomosis with the esophageal veins, rectal venous plexus, and superficial abdominal veins. The portal venous blood traverses the liver and drains into the inferior vena cava via the hepatic veins.

The portal veins become smaller as they progress from the porta hepatis. Large radicles situated near or approaching the porta hepatis are portal veins, not hepatic veins.

The right and left portal veins course transversly through the liver. Anatomically, any intraparenchymal segment of the portal venous system lying to the right of the lateral aspect of the inferior vena cava is a branch of the right portal system. The left portal vein has a narrow-caliber trunk and may be seen coursing transversely through the left hepatic lobe from posterior to anterior.

¹Main portal vein
²Right portal vein
³Left portal vein
⁴Hepatic veins
⁵Bile ducts
⁶Hepatic artery

Fig. 113 FORMATION OF THE PORTAL VEIN

Splenic Vein (Fig. 113)

The splenic vein is a tributary of the portal circulation. It begins at the hilum of the spleen as the union of several veins and is then joined by the short gastric and left gastroepiploic veins. It passes to the right within the lienorenal ligament and runs posterior to the pancreas below the splenic artery. It joins the superior mesenteric vein behind the neck of the pancreas to form the portal vein. It is joined by veins from the pancreas and the inferior mesenteric vein.

Superior Mesenteric Vein

The superior mesenteric vein is a tributary of the portal circulation. It begins at the ileocolic junction and runs upward along the posterior abdominal wall within the root of the mesentery of the small intestine and to the right of the superior mesenteric artery. It passes anterior to the third part of the duodenum and posterior to the neck of the pancreas, where it joins the splenic vein to form the portal vein. It also receives tributaries that correspond to the branches of the superior mesenteric artery, joined by the inferior pancreaticoduodenal vein to the right and the right gastroepiploic vein from the right aspect of the greater curvature of the stomach to the left.

Inferior Mesenteric Vein

The inferior mesenteric vein is a tributary of the portal circulation. It begins midway down the anal canal as the superior rectal vein. It runs up the posterior abdominal wall on the left side of the inferior mesenteric artery and the duodenojejunai junction and joins the splenic vein behind the pancreas. It receives many tributaries along its way, including the left colic vein.

Hepatic Veins

The hepatic veins are the largest visceral tributaries of the inferior vena cava. They originate in the liver, and as they increase in caliber, they drain into the inferior vena cava at the level of the diaphragm. The hepatic veins return blood from the liver that was brought to it by the hepatic artery and the portal vein. The hepatic vein has three branches: the right hepatic vein in the right lobe of the liver, the middle hepatic vein in the caudate lobe, and the left hepatic vein in the left lobe of the liver.

Renal Veins

The right renal vein can be seen to flow directly from the renal sinus into the posterolateral aspect of the inferior vena cava. The left renal vein exits the renal sinus and follows a course anterior to the abdominal aorta and posterior to the superior mesenteric artery to enter the medial aspect of the inferior vena cava. Above the entry of the renal veins, the inferior vena cava enlarges to accommodate the increased volume of blood returning from the kidneys.

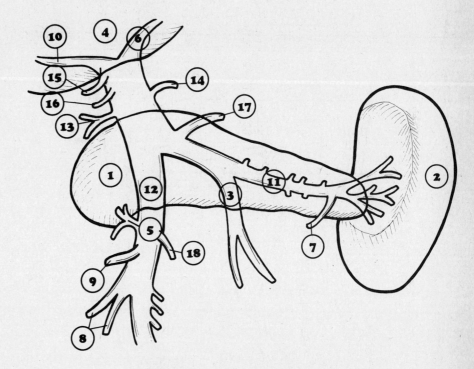

¹Pancreas
²Spleen
³Inferior mesenteric vein
⁴Liver
⁵Inferior pancreaticoduodenal vein
⁶Left branch of the portal vein
⁷Left gastroepiploic vein
⁸Right colic vein
⁹Right gastroepiploic vein
¹⁰Right branch of the portal vein
¹¹Splenic vein
¹²Superior mesenteric vein
¹³Superior pancreaticoduodenal vein
¹⁴Accessory pancreatic vein
¹⁵Cystic vein
¹⁶Right gastric vein (pyloric)

Fig. 114 THORACIC AORTA AND ITS TRIBUTARIES

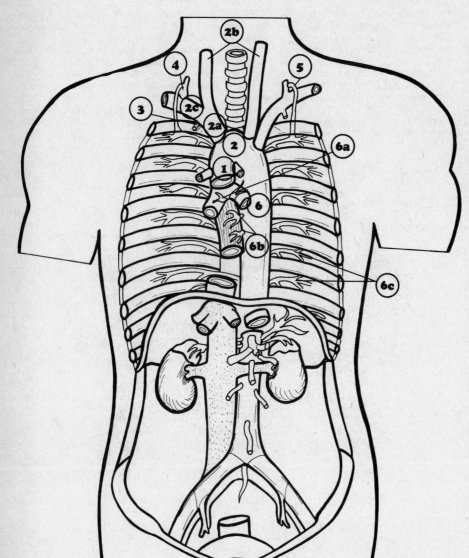

MAIN SYSTEM ARTERIES

Aorta (Figs. 114 and 115)

The systemic circulation leaves the left ventricle of the heart by way of the aorta, the largest artery in the body. The ascending aorta arises from the left ventricle to form the aortic arch. It then arches to the left and curves downward to form the descending aorta. The descending aorta enters the abdomen through the aortic opening of the diaphragm in front of the twelfth thoracic vertebra in the retroperitoneal space. It descends anteriorly to the bodies of the lumbar vertebrae. At the level of the fourth lumbar vertebra it divides into the two common iliac arteries.

The diameter of the aorta is generally between 2 cm and 4 cm. This diameter is fairly uniform throughout its length, with slight variations in contour as it branches to the visceral organs. The aorta has four main branches that supply other visceral organs and the mesentery: the celiac trunk, the superior and inferior mesenteric arteries, and the renal arteries.

The common iliac arteries arise at the bifucation of the aorta and run downward and laterally along the medial border of the right and left psoas muscles. At the level of the sacroiliac joint, each iliac artery bifucates into an external and internal iliac artery.

The external iliac artery runs along the medial border of the psoas, following the pelvic brim. It gives off the inferior epigastric and deep circumflex branches before passing under the inguinal ligament to become the femoral artery.

The internal iliac artery enters the pelvis in front of the sacroiliac joint, at which point it is crossed anteriorly by the ureter. It also divides into anterior and posterior branches to supply the pelvic viscera, peritoneum, buttocks, and sacral canal.

1 Ascending aorta
2 Aortic arch
2a Brachiocephalic artery
2b Common carotid arteries
2c Subclavian artery
3 Internal thoracic artery
4 Costocervical trunk
5 Highest intercostal artery
6 Thoracic (descending) aorta
6a Bronchial arteries
6b Esophageal arteries
6c Posterior intercostal arteries

Fig. 115 ABDOMINAL AORTA AND ITS TRIBUTARIES

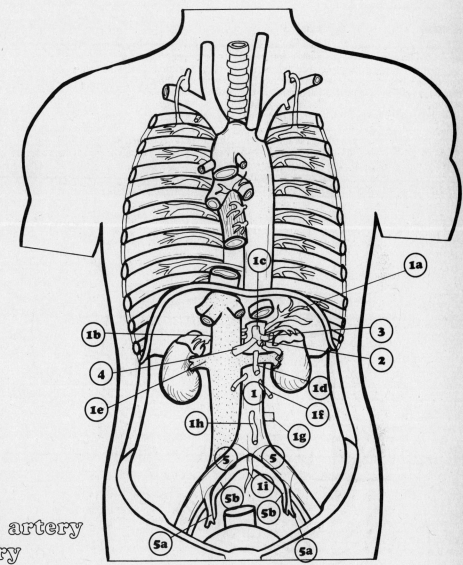

¹Abdominal aorta
¹ᵃInferior phrenic artery
¹ᵇSuprarenal artery
¹ᶜCeliac trunk
¹ᵈSuperior mesenteric artery
¹ᵉRenal artery
¹ᶠTesticular or ovarian artery
¹ᵍLumbar artery
¹ʰInferior mesenteric artery

¹ⁱMiddle sacral artery
²Left gastric artery
³Splenic artery
⁴Hepatic artery
⁵Common iliac arteries
⁵ᵃInternal iliac arteries
⁵ᵇExternal iliac arteries

Fig. 116 CELIAC ARTERY AND ITS BRANCHES

Celiac Trunk (Fig. 116)

The celiac trunk, originating within the first 2 cm of the abdominal aorta, is surrounded by the liver, spleen, inferior vena cava, and pancreas. It immediately branches into the left gastric, splenic, and common hepatic arteries.

The splenic artery is the largest of the three branches of the celiac trunk. From its origin, it takes a somewhat tortuous course horizontally to the left along the upper margin of the pancreas (Fig. 117). Near the splenic hilum, it divides into two branches. The left gastroepi-ploic artery runs caudally into the greater omentum and toward the right gastroepiploic artery. The other branch runs cephalad and divides into the short gastric artery, which supplies the fundus of the stomach, and a number of splenic branches that supply the spleen. Several small branches originate at the splenic artery as it runs along the upper border of the pancreas: the dorsal pancreatic, the great pancreatic, and the caudal pancreatic, among others.

The dorsal pancreatic (or superior pancreatic) artery usually originates from the begining of the splenic artery but may also arise from the hepatic artery, celiac trunk, or aorta. It runs behind and in the substance of the pancreas, dividing into right and left branches. The left branch is the transverse pancreatic artery. The right branch constitutes an anastomotic vessel to the anterior pancreatic arch and also a branch to the uncinate process.

The great pancreatic artery originates from the splenic artery farther to the left and passes downward, dividing into branches that anastomose with the transverse or inferior pancreatic artery.

The caudal pancreatic artery supplies the tail of the pancreas and divides into branches that anastomose with terminal branches of the transverse pancreatic artery.

The transverse pancreatic artery courses behind the body and tail of the pancreas close to the lower pancreatic border. It may originate from or communicate with the superior mesenteric artery.

The common hepatic artery comes off the celiac trunk and courses to the right of the aorta at almost a 90° angle. It courses along the upper border of the pancreatic head, behind the posterior layer of the peritoneal omental bursa, to the upper margin of the superior part of the duodenum, which forms the lower boundary of the epiploic foramen. It ascends into the liver with the hepatic ducts and portal vein. It divides into two main branches: the right hepatic branch, which serves the gallbladder via the cystic artery, and the left hepatic branch, which serves the caudate and left lobes of the liver.

Within the liver parenchyma, the hepatic arterial branches further divide repeatedly into progressively smaller vessels that eventually supply the portal triad.

The head of the pancreas, the duodenum, and parts of the stomach are supplied by the gastroduodenal artery, which arises from the common hepatic artery.

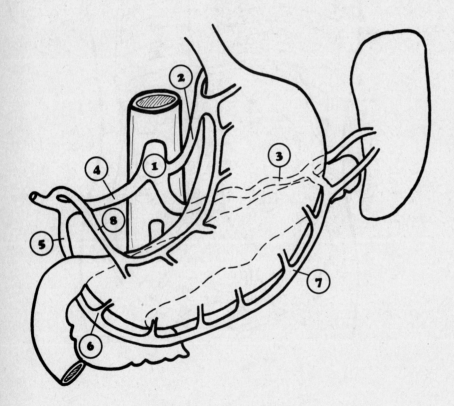

¹Celiac artery
²Left gastric artery
³Splenic artery
⁴Common hepatic artery
⁵Gastroduodenal artery
⁶Right gastroepiploic artery
⁷Left gastroepiploic artery
⁸Right gastric artery

Fig. 117 ANTERIOR VIEW OF THE PANCREAS AND ITS VASCULAR STRUCTURES

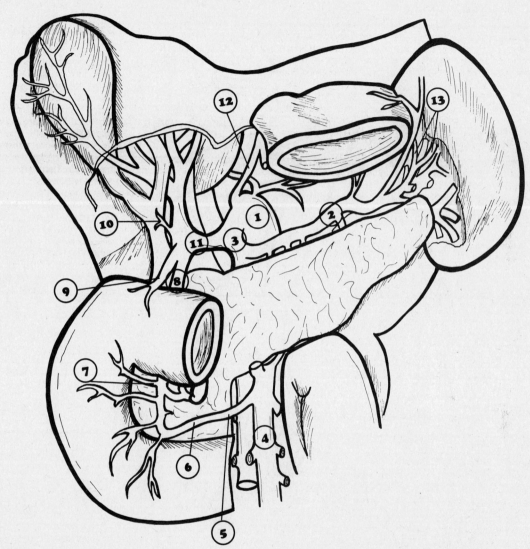

¹Aorta
²Splenic artery
³Celiac trunk
⁴Superior mesenteric artery
⁵Inferior pancreaticoduodenal artery
⁶Anterior inferior pancreaticoduodenal artery
⁷Anterior superior pancreaticoduodenal artery
⁸Gastroduodenal artery
⁹Supraduodenal artery
¹⁰Right gastric artery
¹¹Common hepatic artery
¹²Left gastric artery
¹³Short gastric arteries

Fig. 118 BLOOD SUPPLY TO THE JEJUNUM AND ILEUM*

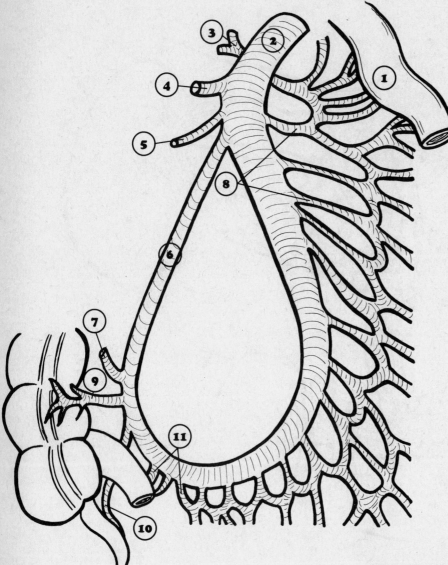

Superior Mesenteric Artery (Fig. 118)

The superior mesenteric artery arises anteriorly from the abdominal aorta approximately 1 cm below the celiac trunk. It runs posterior to the neck of the pancreas, passing over the uncinate process of the pancreatic head anterior to the third part of the duodenum, where it enters the root of the mesentery and colon. It has five main branches: the inferior pancreatic, the duodenal, the colic, the ileocolic, and the intestinal arteries. These branch arteries to the small bowel themselves consist of 10 to 16 branches arising from the left side of the superior mesenteric trunk. They extend into the mesentery, where adjacent arteries unite to form loops, or arcades. Their distribution is to the proximal half of the colon and small intestine.

¹Duodenojejunal flexure
²Superior mesenteric artery
³Inferior pancreaticoduodenal arteries
⁴Middle colic artery
⁵Right colic artery
⁶Ileocolic artery
⁷Ascending branch of ileocolic artery
⁸Intestinal arteries
⁹Cecal arteries
¹⁰Appendicular artery
¹¹Ileal branches of the ileocolic artery

*The ileocolic artery lies at the base of the mesentery of the intestine; the stem of the superior mesenteric artery flows into the mesentery.

Fig. 119 BLOOD SUPPLY OF THE COLON

Inferior Mesenteric Artery (Fig. 119)

The inferior mesenteric artery arises from the anterior abdominal aorta approximately at the level of the third or fourth lumbar veterbra. It proceeds to the left to distribute arterial blood to the descending colon, sigmoid colon, and rectum. It has three main branches: the left colic, sigmoid, and superior rectal arteries.

Renal Arteries

The right and left renal arteries arise anterior to the first lumbar vertebra and inferior to the superior mesenteric artery from the posterolateral or lateral walls of the aorta. They divide into anterior and inferior suprarenal branches.

The right renal artery passes posterior to the inferior vena cava and anterior to the vertebral column in a posterior and slightly caudal direction. The left renal artery has a direct course from the aorta anterior to the psoas to enter the renal sinus.

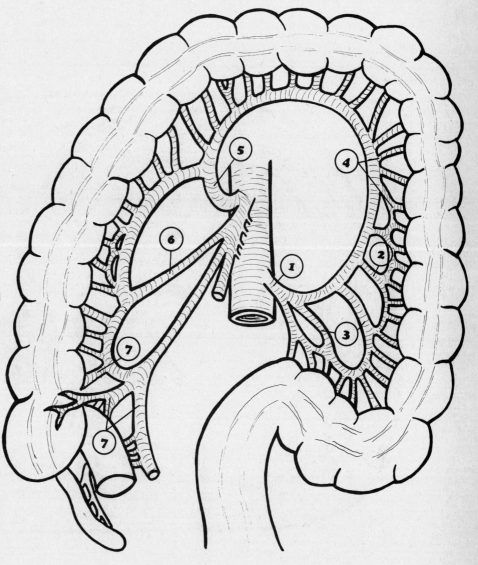

[1] Inferior mesenteric artery
[2] Left colic artery
[3] Sigmoid artery
[4] Marginal arteries
[5] Middle colic artery
[6] Right colic artery
[7] Ileocolic arteries

Fig. 120 SERIAL CROSS SECTION OF THE MAJOR ABDOMINAL VESSELS, LEVEL 1

SERIAL CROSS SECTIONS OF THE MAJOR ABDOMINAL VESSELS (Figs. 120 Through 127)

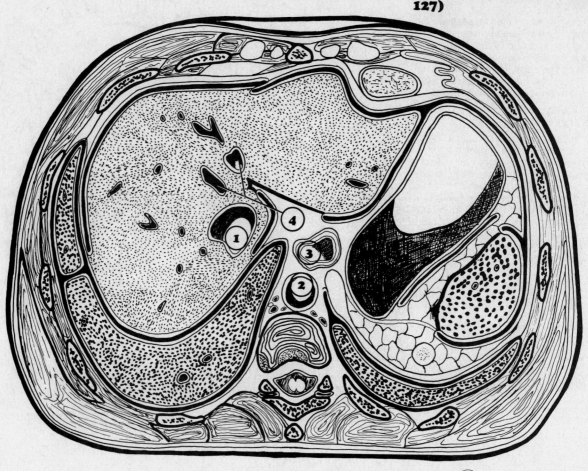

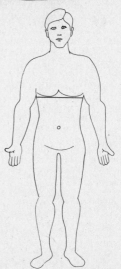

¹Inferior vena cava
²Aorta
³Esophagus
⁴Hepatic veins

Fig. 121 SERIAL CROSS SECTION OF THE MAJOR ABDOMINAL VESSELS, LEVEL 2

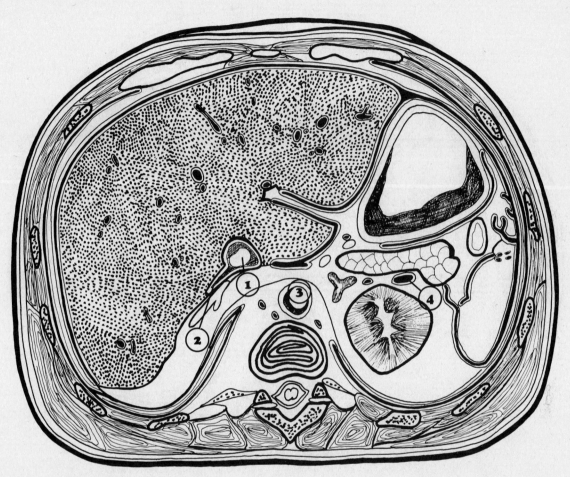

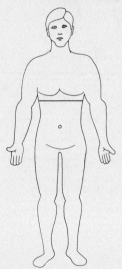

¹Inferior vena cava
²Hepatic vein
³Aorta
⁴Splenic vein

Fig. 122 SERIAL CROSS SECTION OF
THE MAJOR ABDOMINAL
VESSELS, LEVEL 3

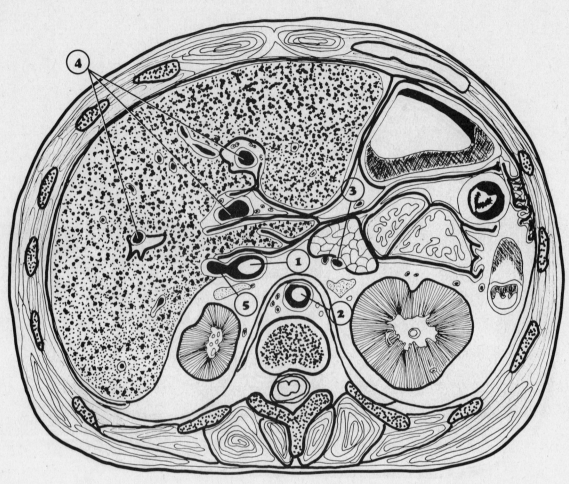

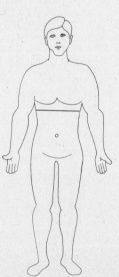

[1]Inferior vena cava
[2]Aorta
[3]Splenic vein
[4]Portal veins
[5]Hepatic vein

Fig. 123 SERIAL CROSS SECTION OF THE MAJOR ABDOMINAL VESSELS, LEVEL 4

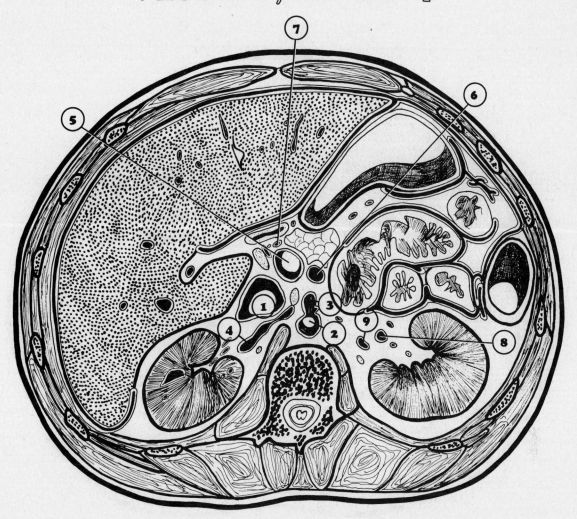

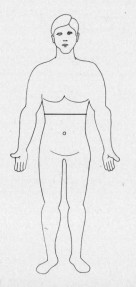

1 Inferior vena cava
2 Aorta
3 Superior mesenteric artery
4 Right renal artery
5 Portal vein
6 Splenic vein
7 Gastroduodenal artery
8 Left renal vein
9 Left renal artery

Fig. 124 SERIAL CROSS SECTION OF
THE MAJOR ABDOMINAL
VESSELS, LEVEL 5

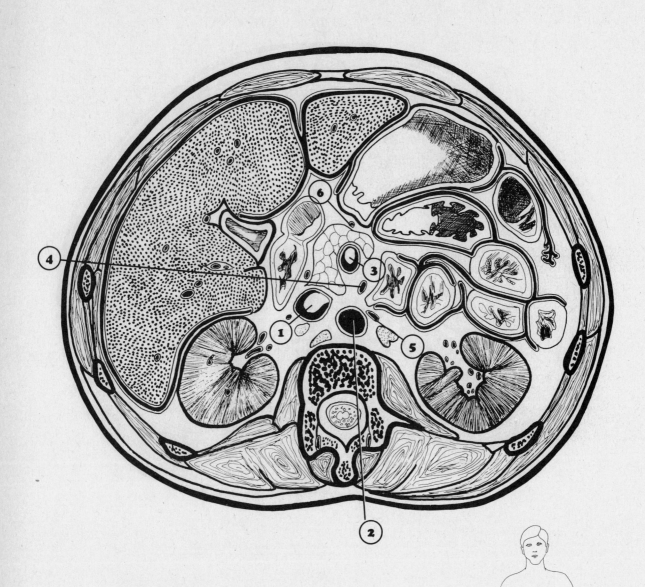

¹Inferior vena cava
²Aorta
³Superior mesenteric
   vein
⁴Superior mesenteric
   artery
⁵Left renal vein
⁶Gastroduodenal artery

Fig. 125 SERIAL CROSS SECTION OF THE MAJOR ABDOMINAL VESSELS, LEVEL 6

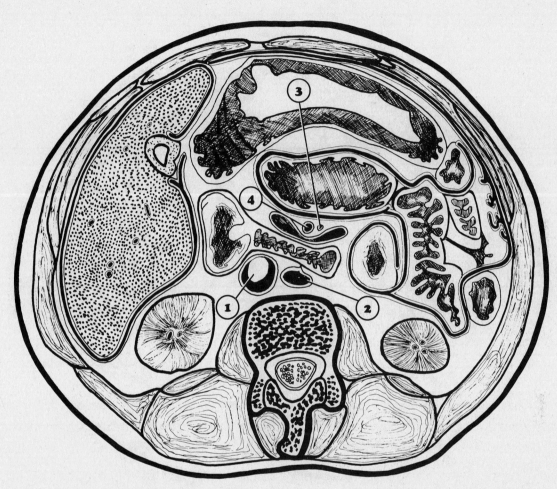

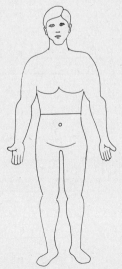

[1]Inferior vena cava
[2]Aorta
[3]Splenic vein
[4]Superior mesenteric artery

Fig. 126 SERIAL CROSS SECTION OF THE MAJOR ABDOMINAL VESSELS, LEVEL 7

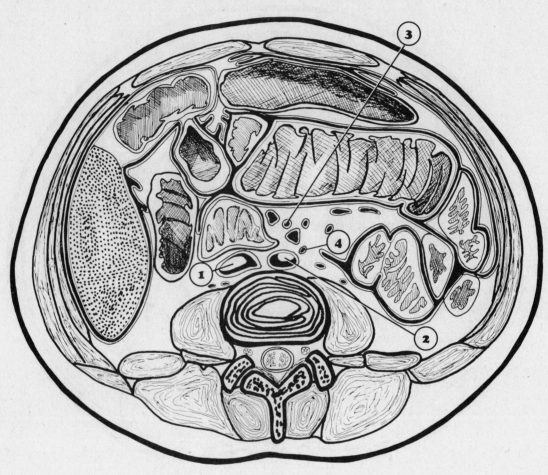

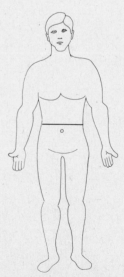

¹Inferior vena cava
²Aorta
³Superior mesenteric
  artery
⁴Inferior mesenteric
  artery

Fig. 127 SERIAL CROSS SECTION OF THE MAJOR ABDOMINAL VESSELS, LEVEL 8

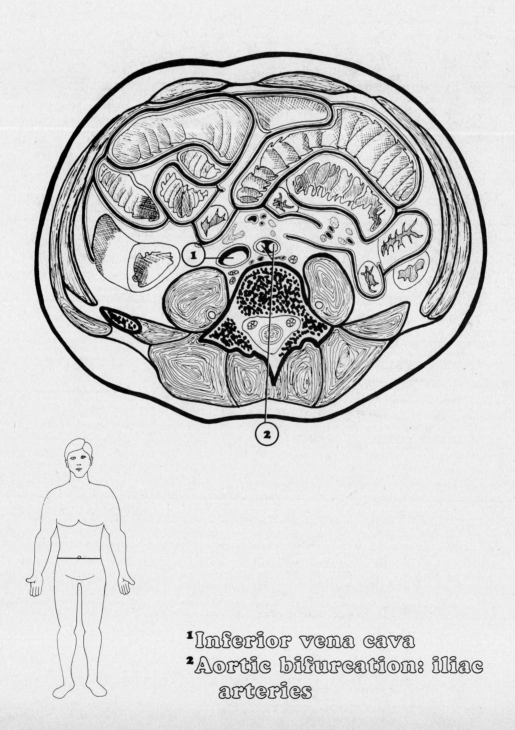

¹Inferior vena cava
²Aortic bifurcation: iliac arteries

Fig. 128 ABDOMINAL SAGITTAL
SECTION, LEVEL 4

**SERIAL SAGITTAL
SECTIONS OF THE MAJOR
ABDOMINAL VESSELS (Figs.
128 Through 135)**

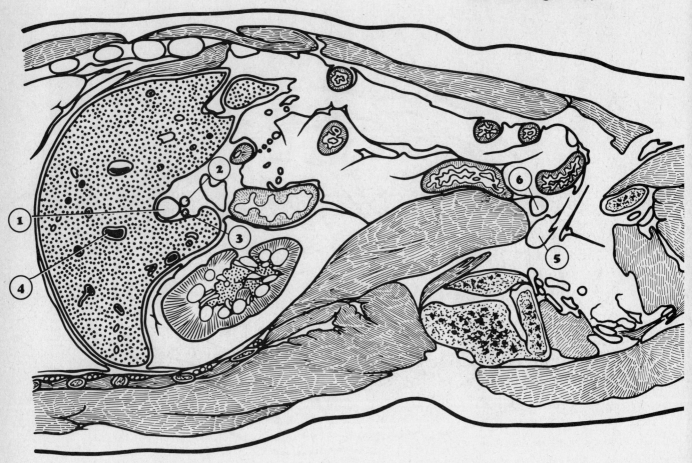

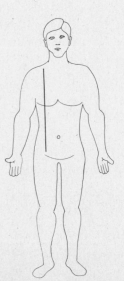

¹Right portal vein
²Hepatic artery
³Common bile duct
⁴Hepatic vein
⁵Right external iliac vein
⁶Right external iliac
   artery

Fig. 129 ABDOMINAL SAGITTAL SECTION, LEVEL 5

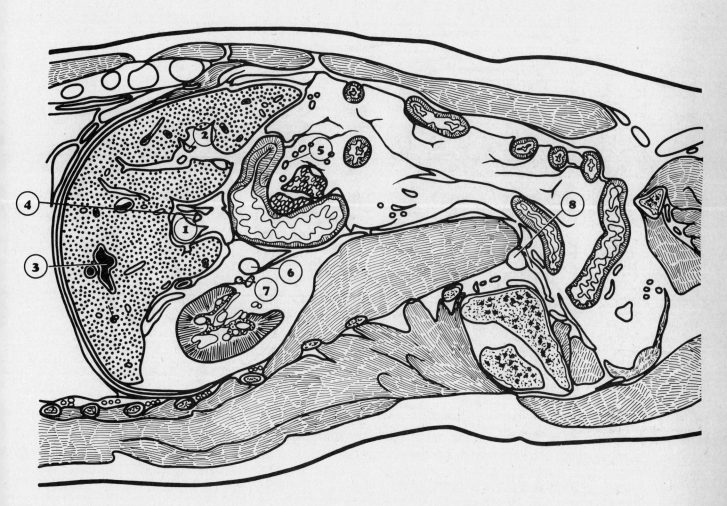

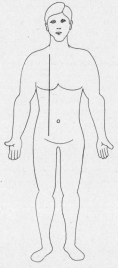

[1]Right portal vein
[2]Left portal vein
[3]Hepatic vein
[4]Cystic duct
[5]Gastroduodenal artery
[6]Right renal vein
[7]Right renal artery
[8]Right external iliac
artery

Fig. 130 ABDOMINAL SAGITTAL SECTION, LEVEL 6

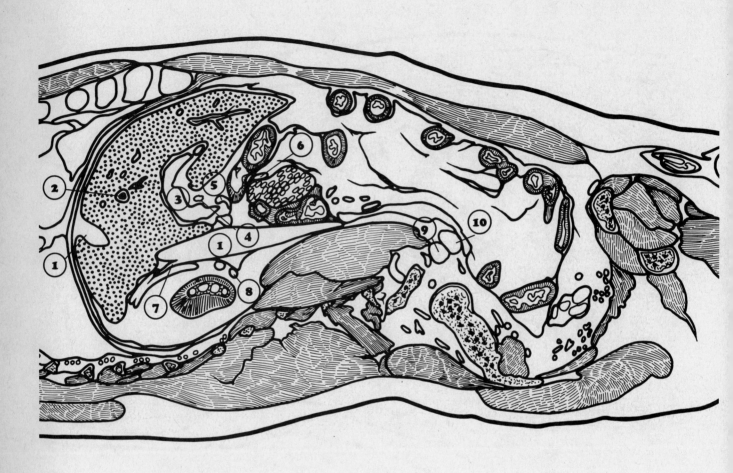

1 Inferior vena cava
2 Hepatic vein
3 Left portal vein
4 Hepatic artery
5 Common bile duct
6 Gastroduodenal artery
7 Right suprarenal vein
8 Right renal artery
9 Right common iliac
    vein
10 Right common iliac
    artery

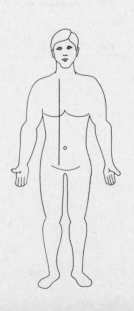

Fig. 131 ABDOMINAL SAGITTAL SECTION, LEVEL 7

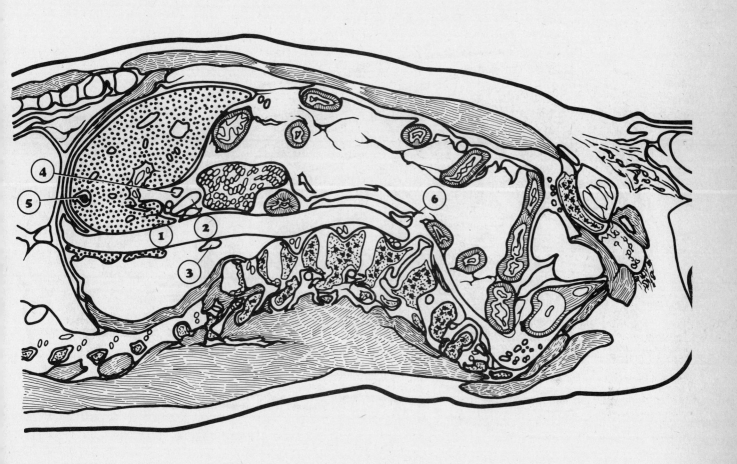

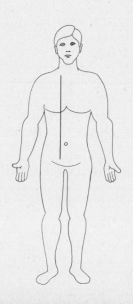

1 Inferior vena cava
2 Portal vein
3 Right renal artery
4 Hepatic artery
5 Hepatic vein
6 Right common iliac artery

Fig. 132 ABDOMINAL SAGITTAL SECTION, LEVEL 8

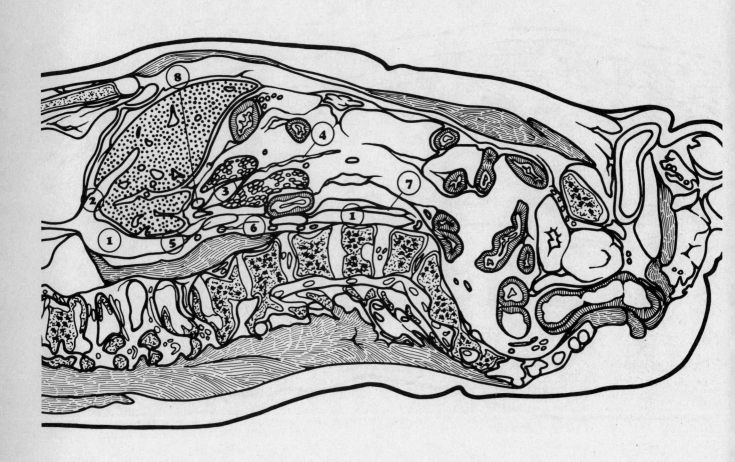

¹Inferior vena cava
²Hepatic vein
³Portal vein
⁴Superior mesenteric
    vein
⁵Left renal vein
⁶Right renal artery
⁷Right common iliac
    artery
⁸Hepatic artery

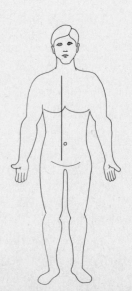

Fig. 133 ABDOMINAL SAGITTAL SECTION, LEVEL 9

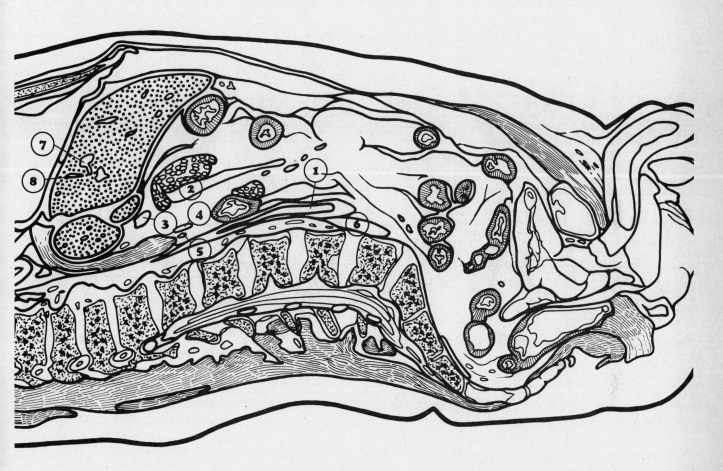

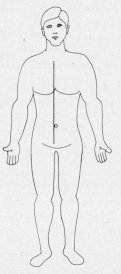

[1] Aorta
[2] Superior mesenteric vein
[3] Hepatic artery
[4] Left renal vein
[5] Right renal artery
[6] Left common iliac vein
[7] Portal vein
[8] Hepatic vein

Fig. 134 ABDOMINAL SAGITTAL SECTION, LEVEL 10

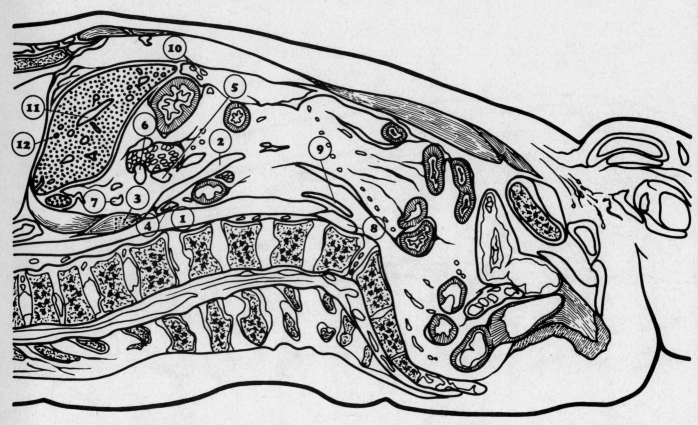

1 Aorta
2 Superior mesenteric artery
3 Celiac trunk
4 Left renal vein
5 Splenic vein
6 Splenic artery
7 Common hepatic artery
8 Left common iliac vein
9 Inferior mesenteric artery
10 Right gastroepiploic artery and vein
11 Portal vein
12 Hepatic vein

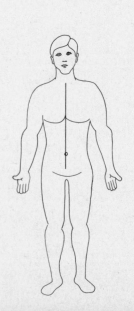

Fig. 135 ABDOMINAL SAGITTAL SECTION, LEVEL 11

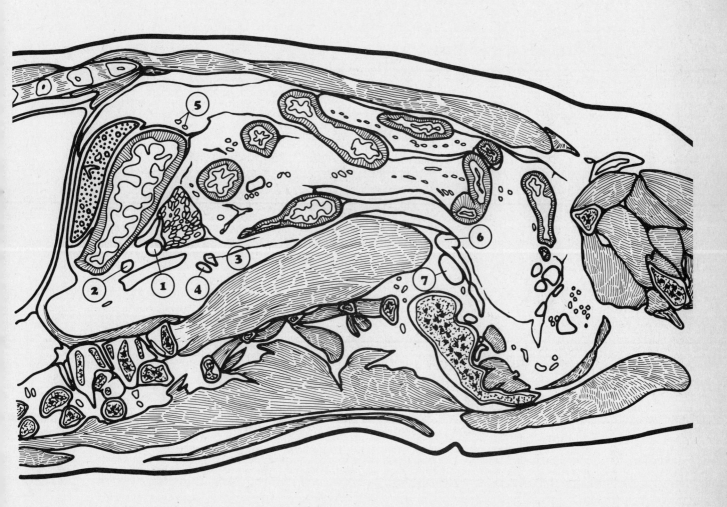

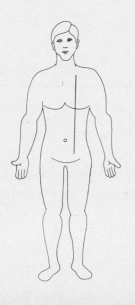

¹Splenic vein
²Splenic artery
³Left renal vein
⁴Left renal artery
⁵Right gastroepiploic
  artery and vein
⁶Left common iliac
  artery
⁷Left common iliac vein

Pancreas

Fig. 136 PANCREAS AND ITS SURROUNDING RELATIONSHIPS

The pancreas is a retroperitoneal gland bounded anteriorly by the stomach and duodenum and posteriorly by the prevertebral vessels (Fig. 136). It is located deep in the epigastrium and left hypochondrium behind the lesser omental sac. The pancreas is generally found in a horizontal-oblique lie, extending from the concavity of the duodenum to the hilum of the spleen. It is approximately 12 cm long and 2 cm thick. The gland is divided into three major areas: head, neck/body, and tail (Figs. 137 and 138).

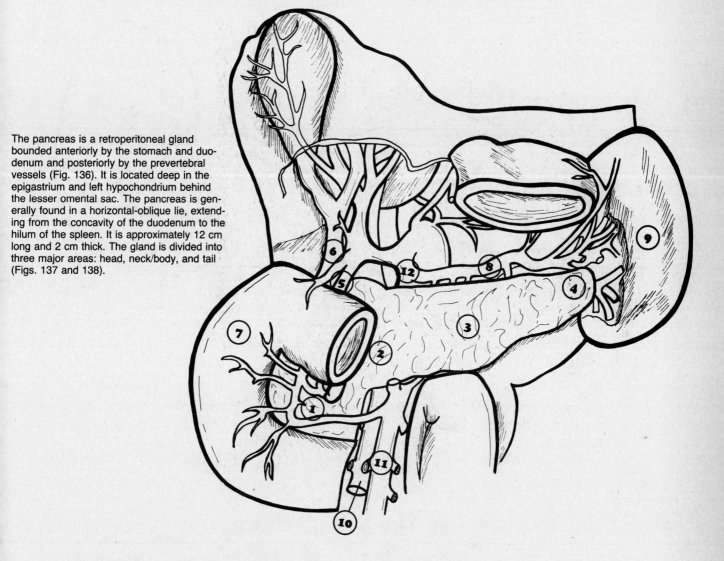

¹Head of the pancreas
²Neck of the pancreas
³Body of the pancreas
⁴Tail of the pancreas
⁵Gastroduodenal artery
⁶Common bile duct
⁷Duodenum

⁸Splenic artery
⁹Spleen
¹⁰Superior mesenteric vein
¹¹Superior mesenteric artery
¹²Celiac axis

Fig. 137 ARTERIAL SUPPLY SURROUNDING THE PANCREAS

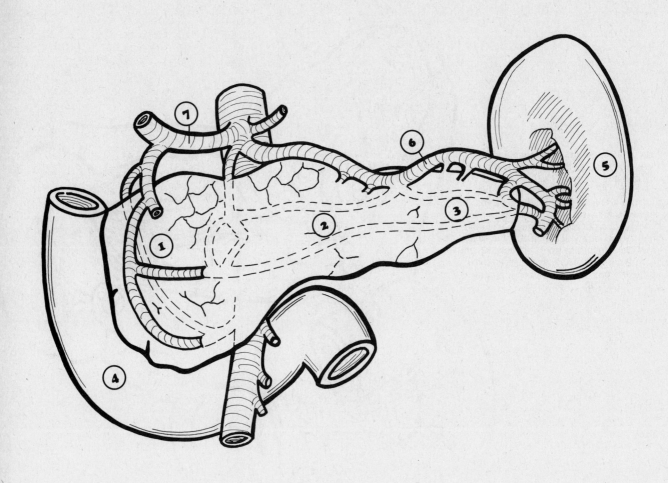

¹Head of the pancreas
²Body of the pancreas
³Tail of the pancreas
⁴Duodenum
⁵Spleen
⁶Splenic artery
⁷Hepatic artery

Fig. 138 PANCREAS AND ITS MAIN ARTERIES

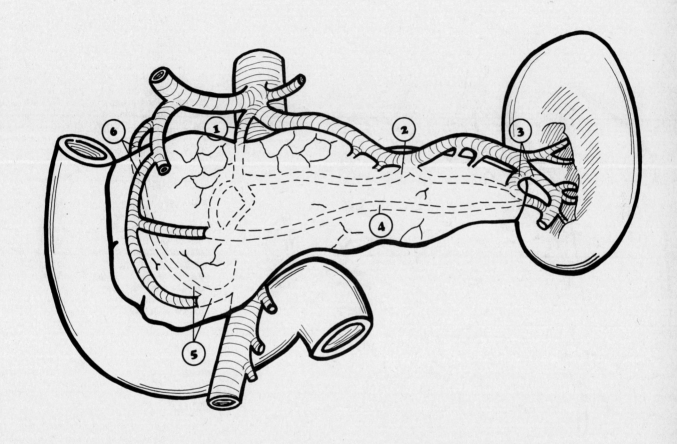

¹Dorsal pancreatic
  artery
²Great pancreatic artery
³Caudal pancreatic
  artery
⁴Inferior pancreatic
  artery

⁵Posterior and
  anterior inferior
  pancreaticoduodenal
  arteries
⁶Posterior and
  anterior superior
  pancreaticoduodenal
  arteries

Fig. 139 BLOOD SUPPLY TO THE PANCREAS AND DUODENUM

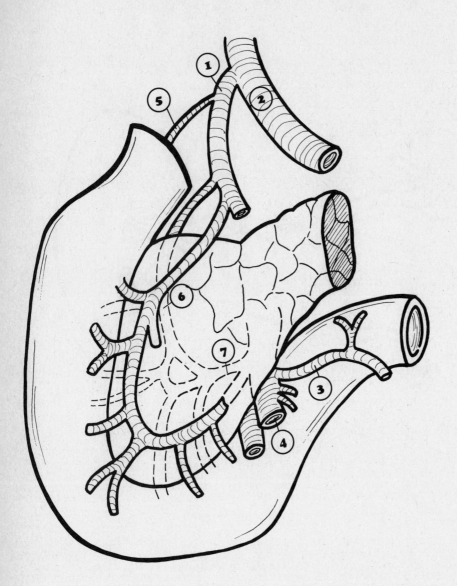

HEAD (Fig. 139)

The head of the pancreas is anterior to the inferior vena cava and left renal vein, inferior to the caudate lobe of the liver and the portal vein, and lateral to the second portion of the duodenum. It lies in the "lap" of the duodenum. These structures pass posterior to the superior mesenteric vessels and antrum of the stomach. The uncinate process is posterior to the superior mesenteric vessels. The common bile duct passes through a groove posterior to the pancreatic head, and the gastroduodenal artery serves as the anterolateral border.

NECK/BODY

The neck/body is the largest part of the gland and lies on an angle from caudal right to cephalad left, posterior to the stomach and anterior to the origin of the portal vein. It rests posteriorly against the aorta, the origin of the superior mesenteric artery, the left renal vessels, the left adrenal glands, and the left kidney. The tortuous splenic artery is usually the superior border of the pancreatic body. The anterior surface is separated by the omental bursa from the posterior wall of the stomach. The inferior surface, below the attachment of the transverse mesocolon, is adjacent to the duodenojejunal junction and the splenic flexure of the colon.

TAIL

The tail of the pancreas lies anterior to the left kidney, close to the spleen and the left colic flexure. The splenic artery forms the anterior border, the splenic vein the posterior border, and the stomach the superoanterior border.

[1] Gastroduodenal artery
[2] Hepatic artery
[3] First jejunal artery
[4] Superior mesenteric artery
[5] Supraduodenal artery
[6] Anterior superior pancreaticoduodenal artery
[7] Posterior and anterior inferior pancreaticoduodenal arteries

Fig. 140 ANTERIOR VIEW OF THE PANCREAS AND DUODENUM

PANCREATIC DUCTS
(Fig. 140)

The duct of Wirsung is a primary duct extending the entire length of the gland. It receives tributaries from lobules at right angles and enters the medial second part of the duodenum with the common bile duct at the ampulla of Vater (guarded by the sphincter of Oddi).

The duct of Santorini is a secondary duct that drains the upper anterior head. It enters the duodenum at the minor papilla approximately 2 cm proximal to the ampulla of Vater.

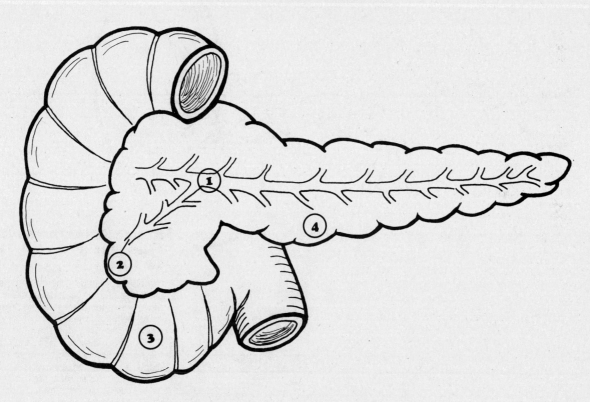

¹Accessory pancreatic duct
²Main pancreatic duct
³Duodenum
⁴Pancreas

Fig. 141 RELATIONSHIP OF THE SPLENIC-PORTAL VEIN TO THE PANCREAS AS VIEWED FROM POSTERIOR

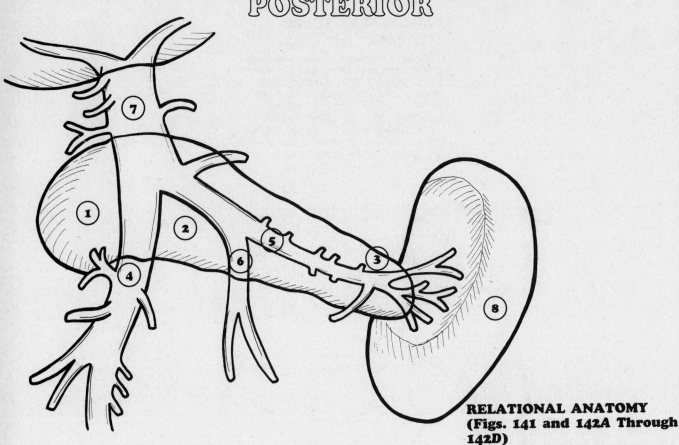

RELATIONAL ANATOMY
(Figs. 141 and 142A Through 142D)

Structures related to the posterior surface include the inferior vena cava, the aorta, the superior mesenteric vessels, the splenic and portal veins, and the common bile duct. The splenic artery and stomach lie along the superior border of the pancreas, and the hilum of the spleen lies in contact with the tail of the gland. The anterior pancreatic surface is bounded by the stomach and the lesser peritoneal cavity, whereas the inferior surface lies along the greater peritoneal cavity.

[1] Head of the pancreas
[2] Body of the pancreas
[3] Tail of the pancreas
[4] Superior mesenteric vein
[5] Splenic vein
[6] Inferior mesenteric vein
[7] Portal vein
[8] Spleen

Fig. 142A CROSS SECTION OF THE PANCREAS AND ITS VASCULAR STRUCTURES, LEVEL XYPHOID — 3 cm

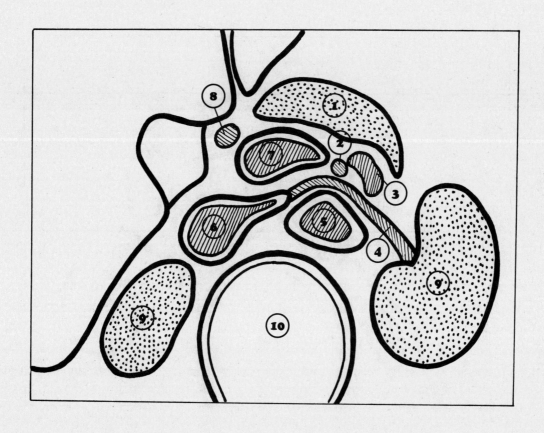

¹Pancreas
²Superior mesenteric artery
³Splenic vein
⁴Left renal vein
⁵Aorta
⁶Inferior vena cava
⁷Portal vein
⁸Gastroduodenal artery
⁹Kidneys
¹⁰Vertebral body

Fig. 142B CROSS SECTION OF THE PANCREAS AND ITS VASCULAR STRUCTURES, LEVEL XYPHOID — 2 cm

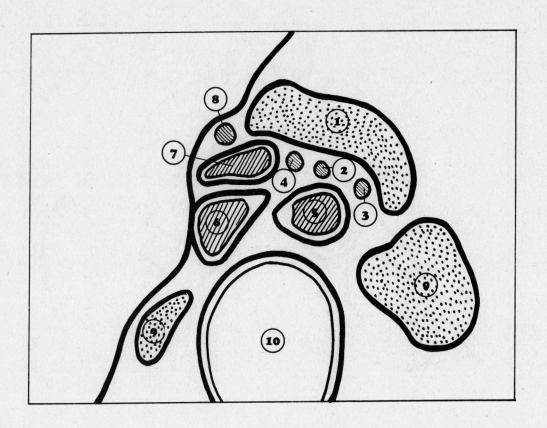

1 Pancreas
2 Superior mesenteric artery
3 Suprarenal vein
4 Left gastric vein
5 Aorta
6 Inferior vena cava
7 Portal vein
8 Gastroduodenal artery
9 Kidneys
10 Vertebral body

Fig. 142C CROSS SECTION OF THE PANCREAS AND ITS VASCULAR STRUCTURES, LEVEL XYPHOID — 1 cm

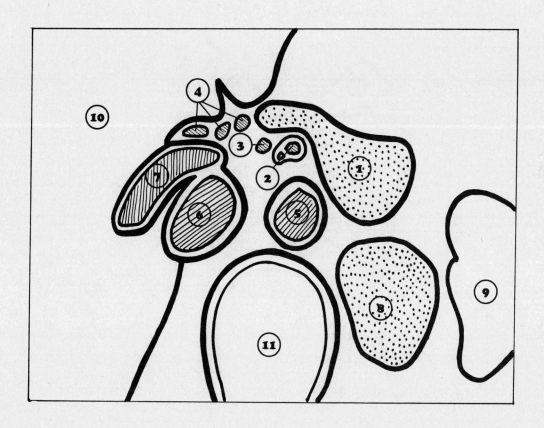

¹Pancreas
²Splenic artery
³Common hepatic artery
⁴Hepatic arteries
⁵Aorta
⁶Inferior vena cava

⁷Portal vein
⁸Kidney
⁹Spleen
¹⁰Liver
¹¹Vertebral body

Fig. 142D CROSS SECTION OF THE PANCREAS AND ITS VASCULAR STRUCTURES, LEVEL XYPHOID

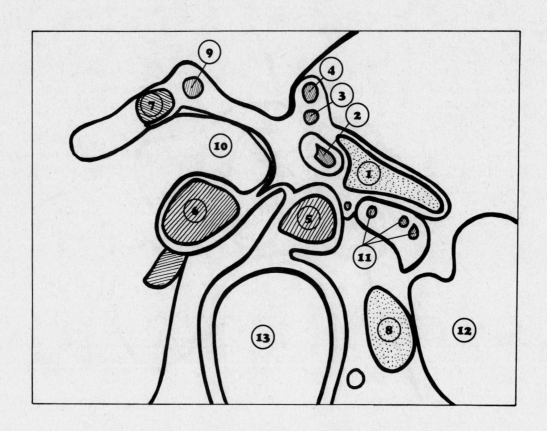

¹Pancreas
²Celiac axis
³Left gastric artery
⁴Left gastric vein
⁵Aorta
⁶Inferior vena cava
⁷Portal vein
⁸Kidney
⁹Hepatic artery
¹⁰Caudate lobe of the liver
¹¹Splenic artery
¹²Spleen
¹³Vertebral body

Fig. 143 CORONAL SECTION OF THE PANCREAS AS VIEWED FROM ANTERIOR

CORONAL SECTIONS OF THE PANCREAS (Figs. 143 and 144)

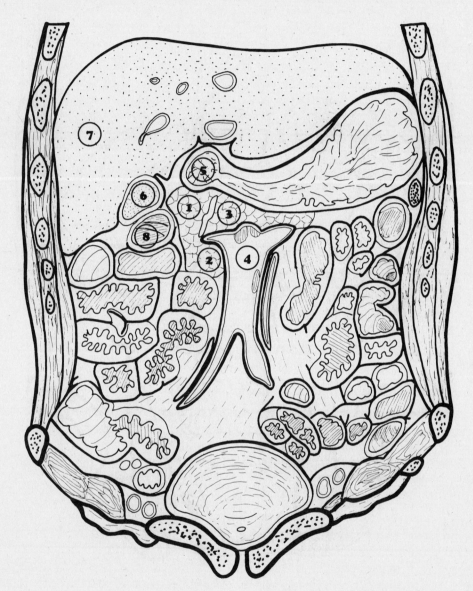

¹Head of the pancreas
²Uncinate process of the pancreas
³Body of the pancreas
⁴Superior mesenteric vein
⁵Duodenum
⁶Gallbladder
⁷Right lobe of the liver
⁸Transverse colon

Fig. 144 CORONAL SECTION OF THE PANCREAS AS VIEWED FROM POSTERIOR

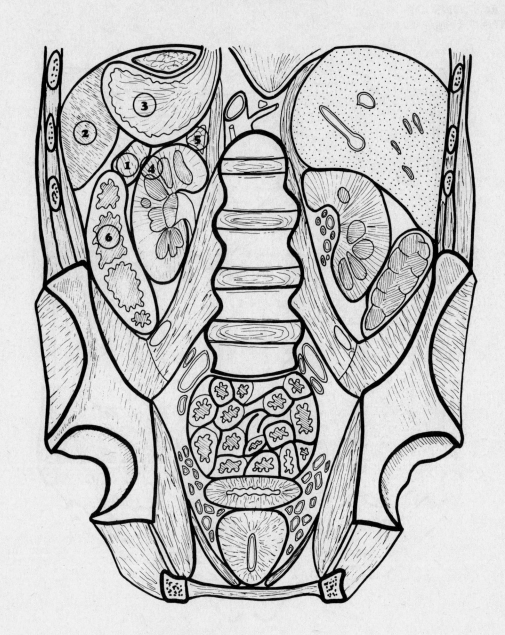

¹Pancreas
²Spleen
³Stomach
⁴Left kidney
⁵Left adrenal gland
⁶Descending colon

Fig. 145 SERIAL CROSS SECTION OF THE PANCREAS, LEVEL 2

SERIAL CROSS SECTIONS OF THE PANCREAS (Figs. 145 Through 148)

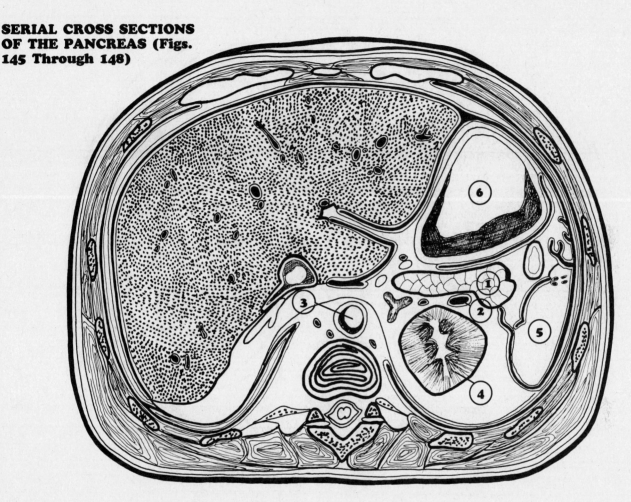

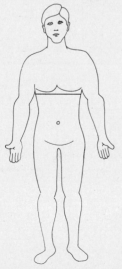

¹Pancreas (tail)
²Splenic vein
³Aorta
⁴Left kidney
⁵Spleen
⁶Stomach

Fig. 146 SERIAL CROSS SECTION OF THE PANCREAS, LEVEL 3

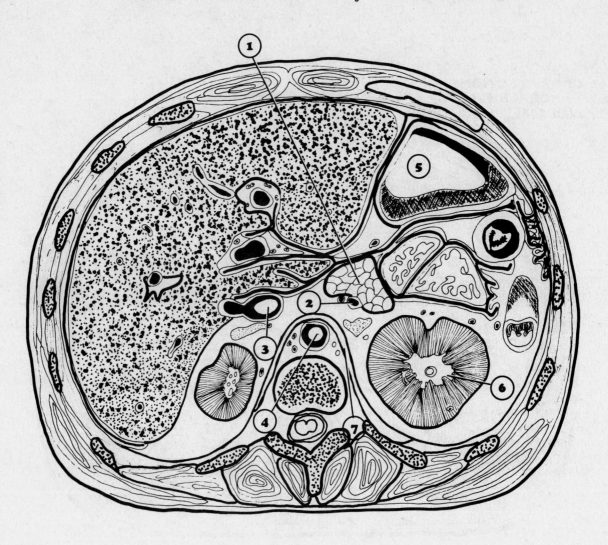

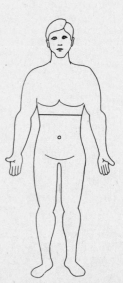

¹Pancreas (body)
²Splenic vein
³Inferior vena cava
⁴Aorta
⁵Stomach
⁶Left kidney
⁷Crus of the diaphragm

Fig. 147 SERIAL CROSS SECTION OF THE PANCREAS, LEVEL 4

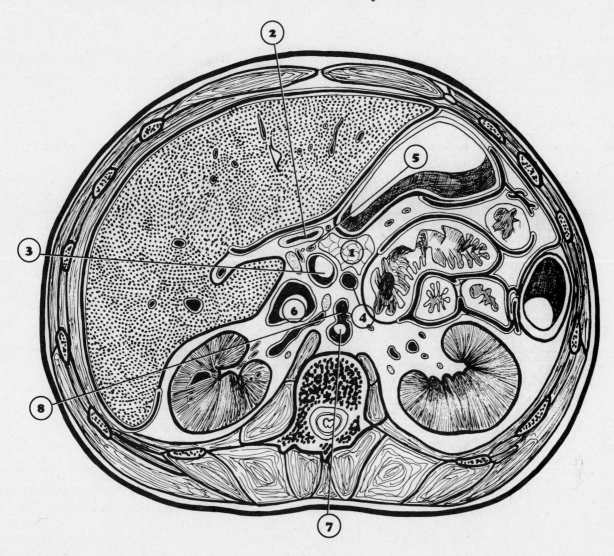

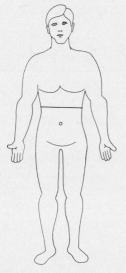

1 Pancreas (body)
2 Duodenum
3 Superior mesenteric vein
4 Splenic vein
5 Gastroduodenal artery
6 Inferior vena cava
7 Aorta
8 Superior mesenteric artery

Fig. 148 SERIAL CROSS SECTION OF THE PANCREAS, LEVEL 5

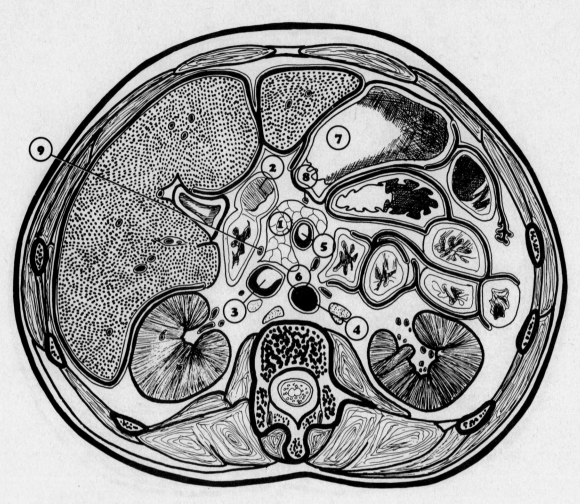

¹Pancreas (head and neck)
²Duodenum
³Inferior vena cava
⁴Aorta
⁵Superior mesenteric vein
⁶Superior mesenteric artery
⁷Stomach
⁸Gastroduodenal artery
⁹Common bile duct

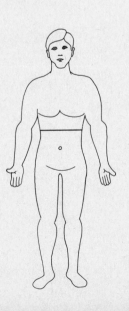

Fig. 149 ABDOMINAL SAGITTAL SECTION, LEVEL 5

SERIAL SAGITTAL SECTIONS OF THE PANCREAS (Figs. 149 Through 156)

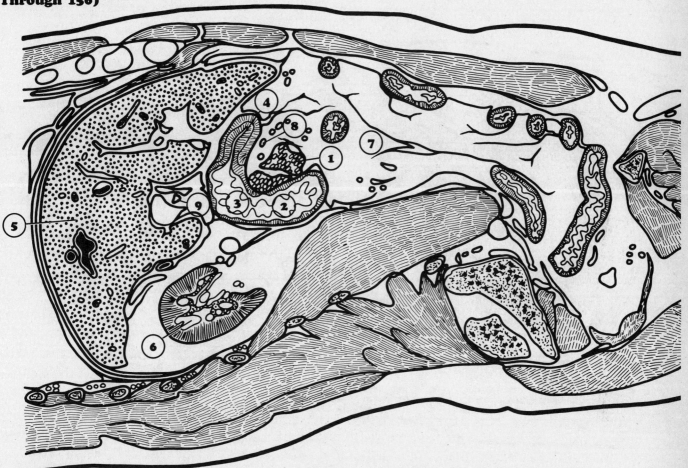

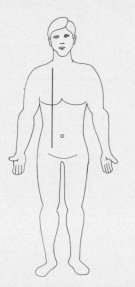

[1] **Head of the pancreas**
[2] **Descending part of the duodenum**
[3] **Superior part of the duodenum**
[4] **Pyloric sphincter**
[5] **Right lobe of the liver**
[6] **Right kidney**
[7] **Mesentery**
[8] **Gastroduodenal artery**
[9] **Cystic duct**

Fig. 150 ABDOMINAL SAGITTAL SECTION, LEVEL 6

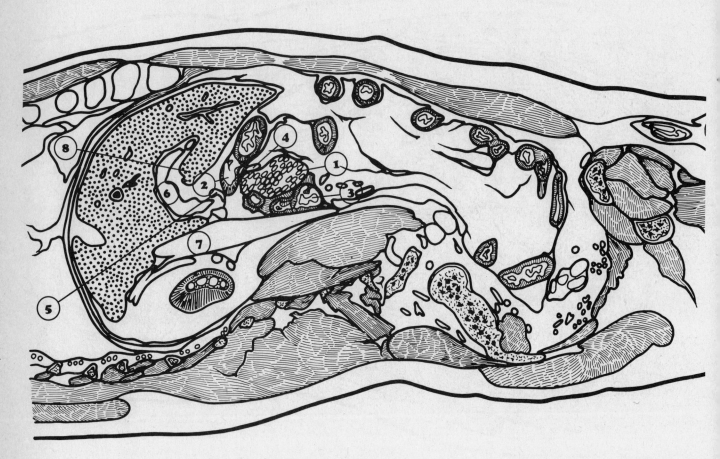

1 Head of the pancreas
2 Descending part of the duodenum
3 Superior part of the duodenum
4 Gastroduodenal artery
5 Common bile duct
6 Left portal vein
7 Inferior vena cava
8 Caudate lobe of the liver

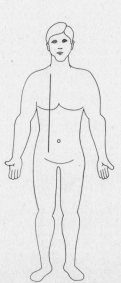

Fig. 151 ABDOMINAL SAGITTAL SECTION, LEVEL 7

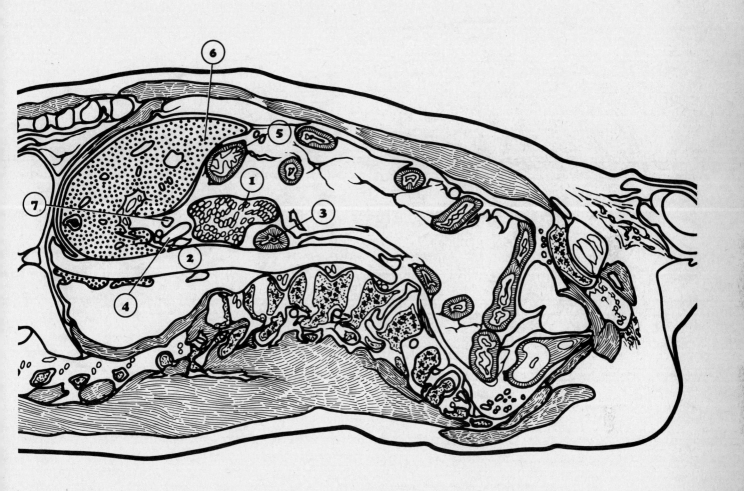

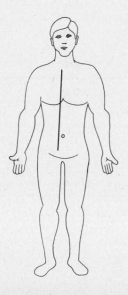

¹Head of the pancreas
²Inferior vena cava
³Horizontal part of the duodenum
⁴Portal vein
⁵Pyloric sphincter
⁶Left lobe of the liver
⁷Hepatic artery

Fig. 152 ABDOMINAL SAGITTAL SECTION, LEVEL 8

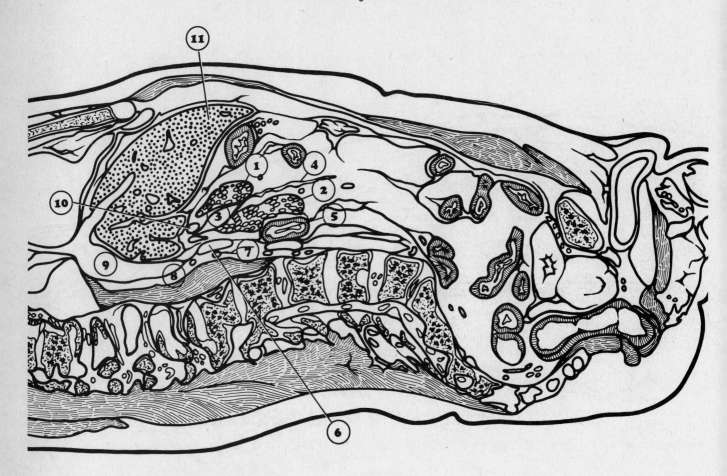

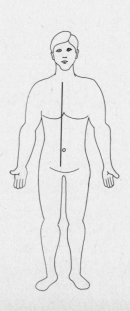

1 Head of the pancreas
2 Uncinate process
3 Portal vein
4 Superior mesenteric vein
5 Horizontal part of the duodenum
6 Left renal vein
7 Right renal artery
8 Crus of the diaphragm
9 Inferior vena cava
10 Hepatic artery
11 Left lobe of the liver

Fig. 153 ABDOMINAL SAGITTAL SECTION, LEVEL 9

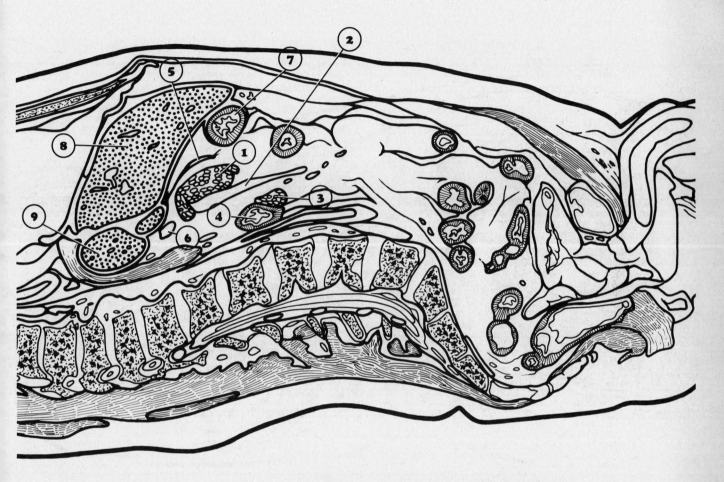

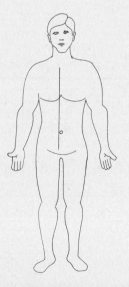

[1]Body of the pancreas
[2]Superior mesenteric vein
[3]Uncinate process of the pancreas
[4]Horizontal part of the duodenum
[5]Lesser sac
[6]Hepatic artery
[7]Pyloric antrum
[8]Left lobe of the liver
[9]Caudate lobe of the liver

Fig. 154 ABDOMINAL SAGITTAL SECTION, LEVEL 10

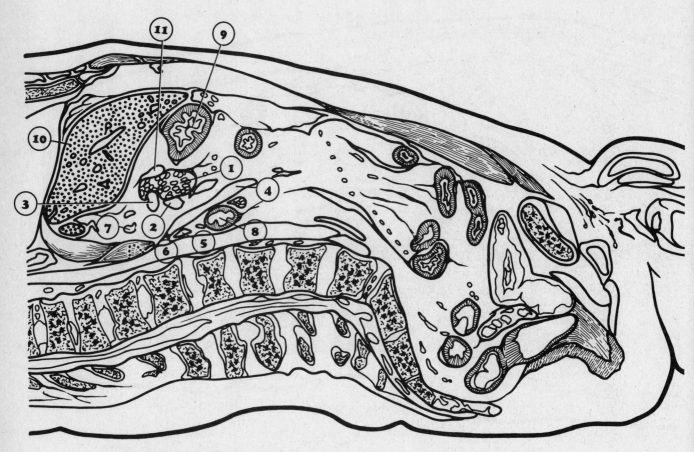

1 Body of the pancreas
2 Splenic vein
3 Splenic artery
4 Superior mesenteric artery
5 Left renal vein
6 Aorta
7 Common hepatic artery
8 Horizontal part of the duodenum
9 Stomach
10 Left lobe of the liver
11 Lesser sac

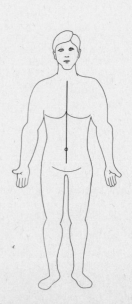

Fig. 155 ABDOMINAL SAGITTAL SECTION, LEVEL 11

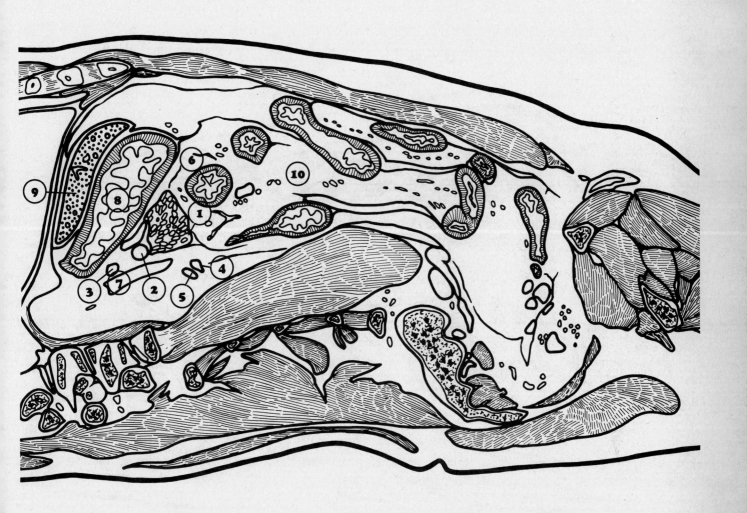

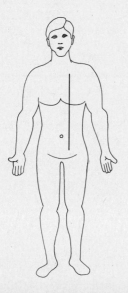

1 Body of the pancreas
2 Splenic vein
3 Splenic artery
4 Left renal vein
5 Left renal artery
6 Ascending part of the duodenum
7 Left suprarenal gland
8 Body of the stomach
9 Left lobe of the liver
10 Mesentery

Fig. 156 ABDOMINAL SAGITTAL SECTION, LEVEL 12

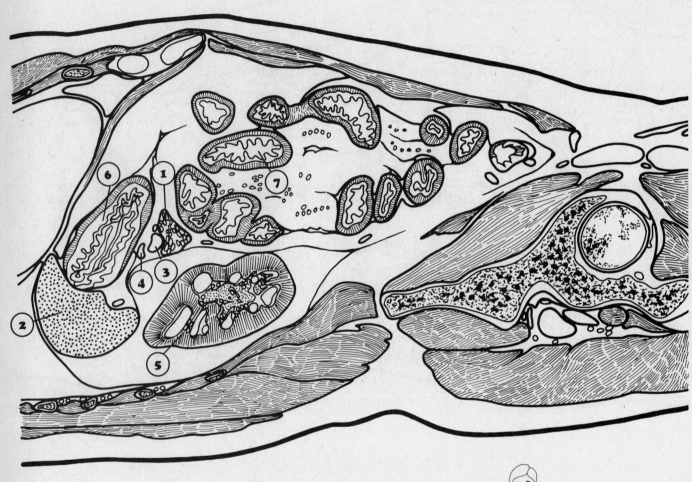

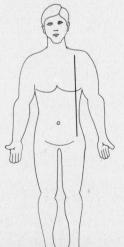

¹Tail of the pancreas
²Spleen
³Splenic vein
⁴Splenic artery
⁵Left kidney
⁶Fundus of the stomach
⁷Small bowel

Spleen

Fig. 157 RELATIONSHIP OF SPLEEN TO ADJACENT STRUCTURES

The spleen is an intraperitoneal organ covered with peritoneum over its entire extent except for a small area at the hilum. The spleen lies in the left hypochondrium, with its axis along the shaft of the tenth rib (Figs. 157 and 158). Its lower pole extends forward as far as the midaxillary line. It is of variable size and shape but is generally considered to be ovoid, with a convex superior and a concave inferior surface. The ends of the spleen are called its posterior and anterior extremities and its borders are superior and inferior.

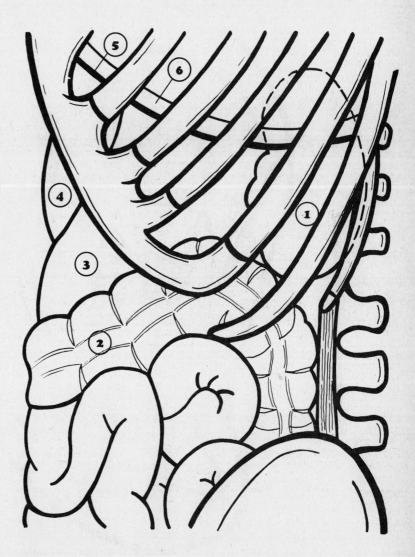

¹Spleen
²Transverse colon
³Stomach
⁴Liver
⁵Diaphragm
⁶Costodiaphragmatic
recess

167

Fig. 158 SPLEEN

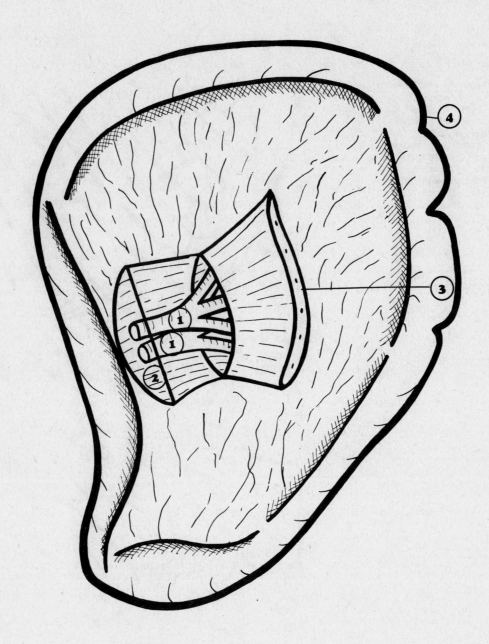

¹Splenic vessels
²Lienorenal ligaments
³Gastrosplenic omentum
⁴Notched anterior
   border

Fig. 159 SPLEEN AND ITS SURROUNDING STRUCTURES

RELATIONAL ANATOMY

Anterior to the spleen lies the stomach, the tail of the pancreas, and the left colic flexure (Fig. 159). The left kidney lies along its medial border. Posteriorly the diaphragm, left pleura, left lung, and ninth, tenth, and eleventh ribs are in contact with the spleen.

Blood is supplied by the splenic artery, which immediately divides into six branches after entering the splenic hilum (Figs. 160 and 161).

The splenic vein leaves the splenic hilum and joins the superior mesenteric vein to form the portal vein (Fig. 162).

The lymph vessels emerging from the hilum pass through a few lymph nodes along the course of the splenic artery and drain into the celiac nodes. The nerves to the spleen accompany the splenic artery and are derived from the celiac plexus.

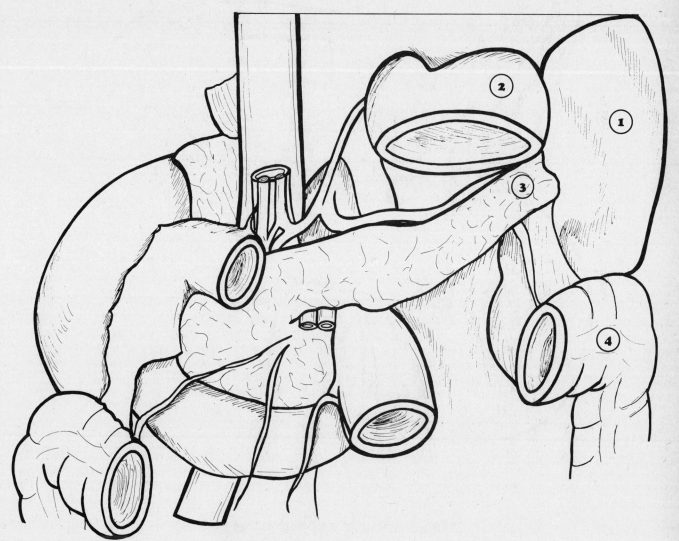

¹Spleen
²Stomach
³Tail of the pancreas
⁴Descending colon

169

Fig. 160 SPLEEN AND ITS ARTERIAL SUPPLY

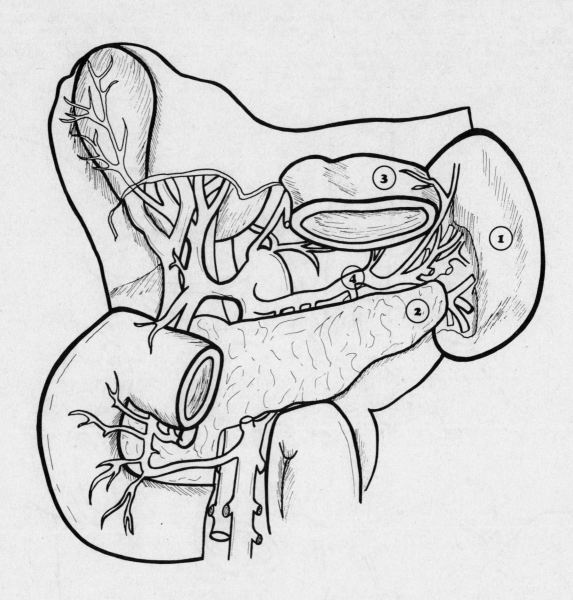

¹Spleen
²Tail of the pancreas
³Stomach
⁴Splenic artery

Fig. 161 ARTERIAL SUPPLY TO THE SPLEEN

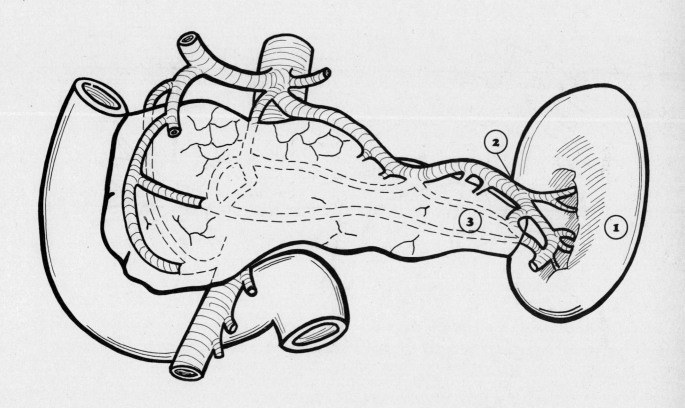

[1]Spleen
[2]Splenic artery
[3]Tail of the pancreas

Fig. 162 SPLEEN AS VIEWED FROM POSTERIOR

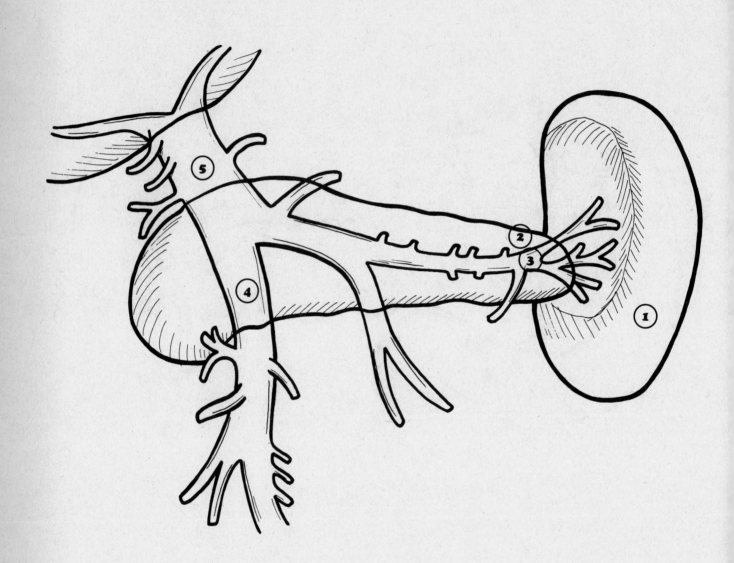

[1]Spleen
[2]Tail of the pancreas
[3]Splenic vein
[4]Superior mesenteric
  vein
[5]Portal vein

Fig. 163 CORONAL VIEW OF THE SPLEEN AS VIEWED FROM POSTERIOR

CORONAL SECTION OF THE SPLEEN (Fig. 163)

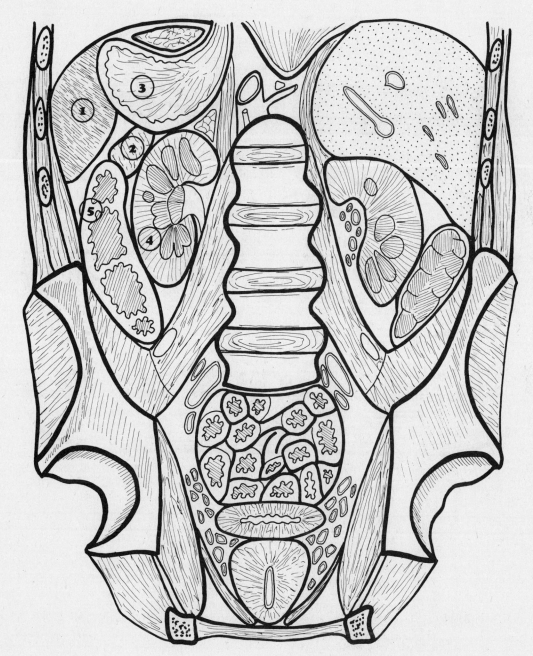

¹Spleen
²Tail of the pancreas
³Stomach

⁴Left kidney
⁵Descending colon

Fig. 164 CROSS SECTION OF THE SPLEEN, LEVEL 1

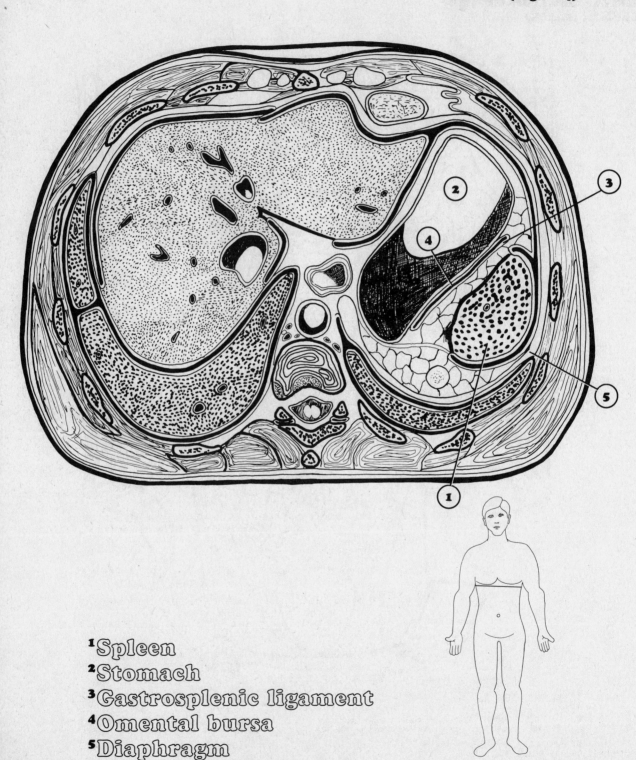

¹Spleen
²Stomach
³Gastrosplenic ligament
⁴Omental bursa
⁵Diaphragm

Fig. 165 ABDOMINAL SAGITTAL SECTION, LEVEL 12

SAGITTAL SECTION OF THE SPLEEN (Fig. 165)

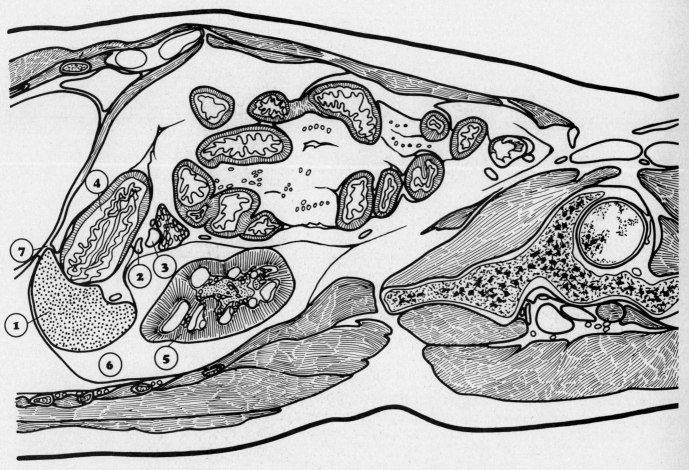

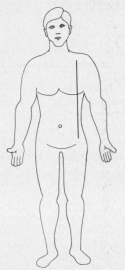

1. Spleen
2. Splenic artery
3. Splenic vein
4. Fundus of the stomach
5. Left kidney
6. Perirenal fat
7. Diaphragm

Retroperitoneal Space

Fig. 166A TRANSVERSE SECTION OF THE ABDOMEN THROUGH THE EPIPLOIC FORAMEN

The retroperitoneal space is the area between the posterior portion of the parietal peritoneum and the posterior abdominal wall muscles (Figs. 166A and 166B). It extends from the diaphragm to the pelvis. Laterally the boundaries extend to the extraperitoneal fat planes within the confines of the transversalis fascia, and medially the space encloses the great vessels.

It is subdivided into three areas: the perinephric space (or fascia of Gerota), the anterior paranephric space, and the posterior paranephric space. The perinephric space surrounds the kidney and the perinephric fat. The anterior paranephric space includes the extraperitoneal surfaces of the gut and pancreas. The iliopsoas muscle, fat, and other soft tissues are within the posterior paranephric space.

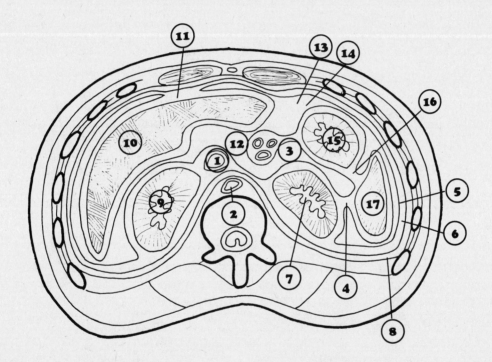

¹Inferior vena cava
²Aorta
³Lesser sac
⁴Lienorenal ligament
⁵Peritoneum
⁶Subserous fascia
⁷Left kidney
⁸Diaphragm
⁹Right kidney
¹⁰Liver
¹¹Falciform ligament
¹²Epiploic foramen
¹³Greater sac
¹⁴Lesser omentum
¹⁵Stomach
¹⁶Gastrolienal ligament
¹⁷Spleen

Fig. 166B TRANSVERSE SECTION OF THE ABDOMINAL CAVITY SHOWING THE REFLECTIONS OF THE PERITONEUM

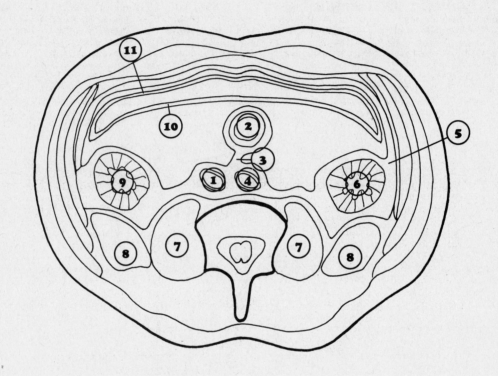

¹Inferior vena cava
²Small intestine
³Mesentery of the small intestine
⁴Aorta
⁵Peritoneum
⁶Descending colon
⁷Psoas major muscle
⁸Quadratus lumborum muscle

⁹Ascending colon
¹⁰Posterior layers of the greater omentum*
¹¹Anterior layers of the greater omentum*

*There is generally no space between the anterior and posterior layers of the greater omentum; they are usually fused together.

Fig. 167 ANTERIOR RELATIONSHIPS OF THE KIDNEYS (STOMACH AND LIVER REMOVED)

KIDNEYS

The kidneys lie on the psoas and quadratus lumborum muscles in the retroperitoneal space under cover of the costal margin. The right kidney lies slightly lower than the left owing to the right lobe of the liver. The left kidney contacts the spleen, pancreas, colon, and jejunum, and the superiomedial pole holds the adrenal gland. The right kidney contacts the liver, colon, and adrenal gland (Fig. 167).

The kidneys are protected posteriorly by the eleventh and twelfth ribs. The inferior poles are not well protected except for that provided by the quadratus lumborum muscle. On the medial surface of the kidney are the hilum, the point of exit of the renal vein, and the point of entrance of the renal artery (Figs. 168 and 169). The renal pelvis is also at the hilum and forms the ureter, which narrows to run posteriorly into the bladder.

The kidneys are approximately 12 cm long, 2.5 cm to 3 cm thick, and 4 cm to 5 cm wide.

The kidney is surrounded by a fibrous capsule, called the true capsule, which is closely applied to the renal cortex (Fig. 170). Outside this capsule is a covering of perinephric fat. The perinephric fascia surrounds the perinephric fat and encloses the kidney and adrenal glands. The renal fascia (Gerota's fascia) surrounds the true capsule and the perinephric fat.

The ureter is 25 cm long and resembles the esophagus in having three constrictions along its course: (1) where it joins the kidney, (2) where it is kinked as it crosses the pelvic brim, and (3) where it pierces the bladder wall (Fig. 171). The pelvis of the ureter is funnel shaped at its upper end. It lies within the hilum of the kidney and receives the major calyces. The ureter emerges from the hilum and runs downward along the psoas, which separates it from the tips of the transverse processes of the lumbar vertebrae. It enters the pelvis by crossing the bifurcation of the common iliac artery in front of the sacroiliac joint. It then runs along the lateral wall of the pelvis to the region of the ischial spine and turns forward to enter the lateral angle of the bladder.

On the medial border of each kidney is the renal hilum, which contains the renal vein, two branches of the renal artery, the ureter, and the third branch of the renal artery.

The kidney is composed of an internal medullary portion and an external cortical substance (Figs. 172 and 173). The medullary substance consists of a series of eight to 18 striated conical masses, called the renal pyramids. Their bases are directed toward the outer circumference of the kidney. Their apices converge toward the renal sinus, where their prominent papillae project into the lumina of the minor calyces.

Within the kidney's upper, expanded end (or pelvis), the ureter divides into two or three major calyces, each of which divides into two or three minor calyces. The four to 13 minor calyces are cup-shaped tubes that usually come into contact with at least one renal papilla. The minor calyces unite to form two or three short tubes, the major calyces; these, in turn, unite to form a funnel-shaped sac, the renal pelvis. Spirally arranged muscles surround the calyces and may exert a milking action on these tubes, aiding in the flow of urine into the renal pelvis. As the renal pelvis leaves the renal sinus, it rapidly becomes smaller and ultimately merges with the ureter.

The kidney is supplied with blood by the renal arteries. The arteries divide into two primary branches, a larger anterior branch and a posterior branch. The arteries finally break down into minute arterioles and are called interlobar arteries. In the portion of the kidney between the cortex and medulla, these arteries are called arcuate arteries.

The renal veins also break down into these categories. Five or six veins join to form the renal vein, which merges from the hilum anterior to the renal artery. The renal vein drains into the inferior vena cava. Further breakdown of the veins and arteries leads to the afferent and efferent glomerular vessels.

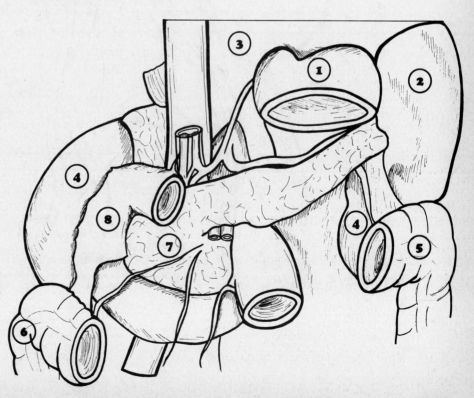

¹Stomach
²Spleen
³Diaphragm
⁴Kidney
⁵Descending colon
⁶Ascending colon
⁷Pancreas
⁸Duodenum

Fig. 168 KIDNEYS, SUPRARENAL GLANDS, AND VASCULAR STRUCTURES

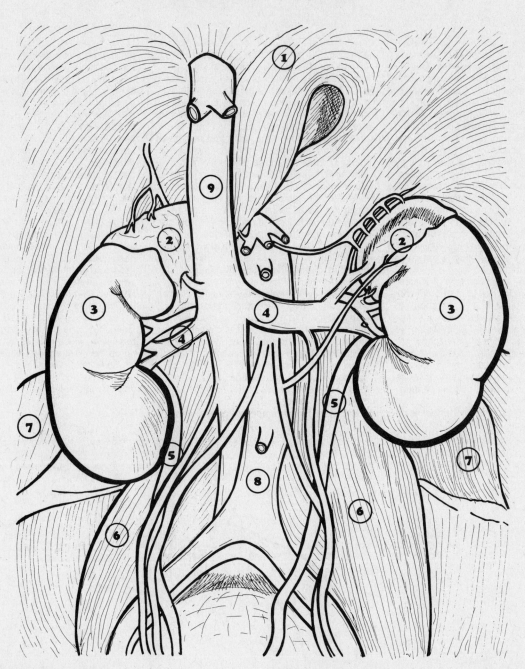

¹Diaphragm
²Suprarenal gland
³Kidney
⁴Renal vein
⁵Ureter

⁶Psoas major muscle
⁷Quadratus lumborum
    muscle
⁸Aorta
⁹Inferior vena cava

Fig. 169 KIDNEYS AND THEIR VASCULAR RELATIONSHIPS

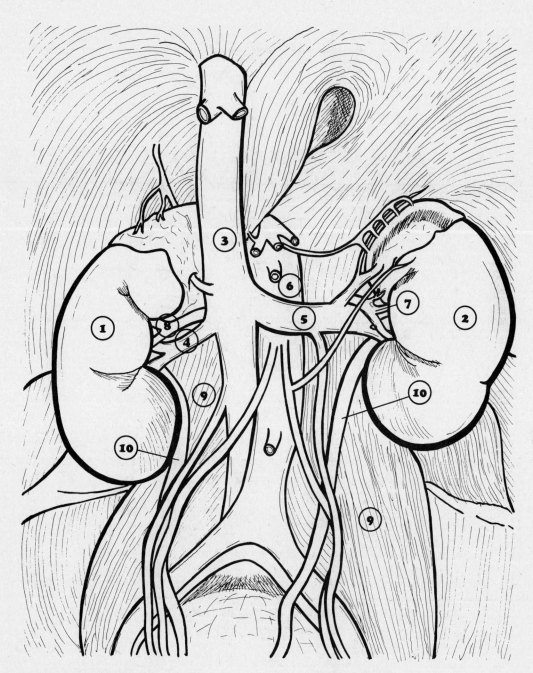

[1] Right kidney	[6] Aorta
[2] Left kidney	[7] Left renal artery
[3] Inferior vena cava	[8] Right renal artery
[4] Right renal vein	[9] Psoas muscle
[5] Left renal vein	[10] Ureter

Fig. 170 KIDNEY

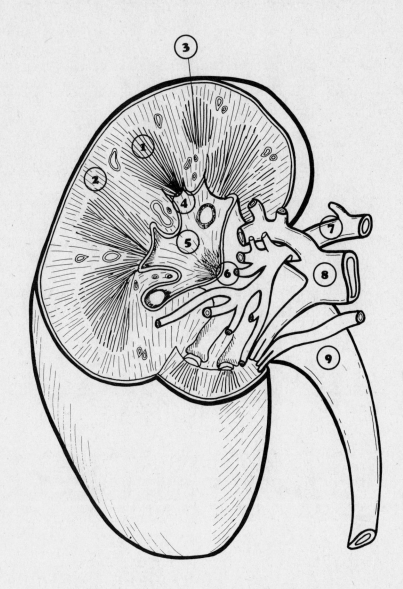

[1] Renal medulla
(pyramid)
[2] Renal cortex
[3] Renal papilla
[4] Minor calyx
[5] Major calyx
[6] Renal pelvis
[7] Renal artery
[8] Renal vein
[9] Ureter

Fig. 171 BLOOD SUPPLY OF THE URETER (MALE)

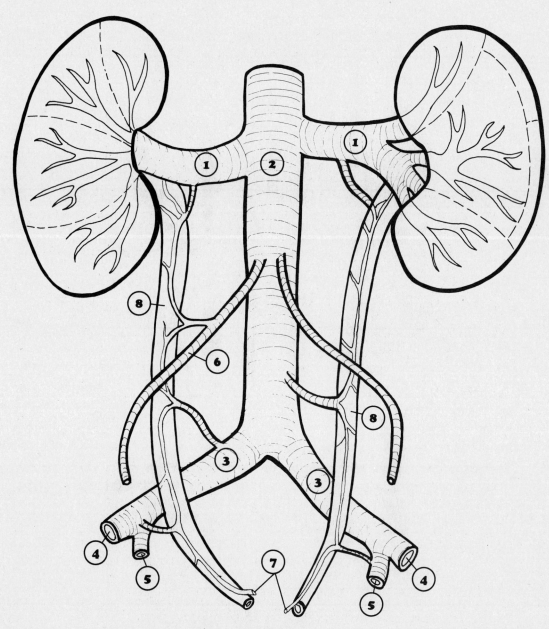

1 Renal artery
2 Aorta
3 Common iliac artery
4 External iliac artery
5 Internal iliac artery
6 Testicular artery
7 Inferior vesical and
   uterine arteries
8 Ureter

Fig. 172 ANATOMICAL STRUCTURES RELATED TO THE ANTERIOR SURFACES OF THE KIDNEYS

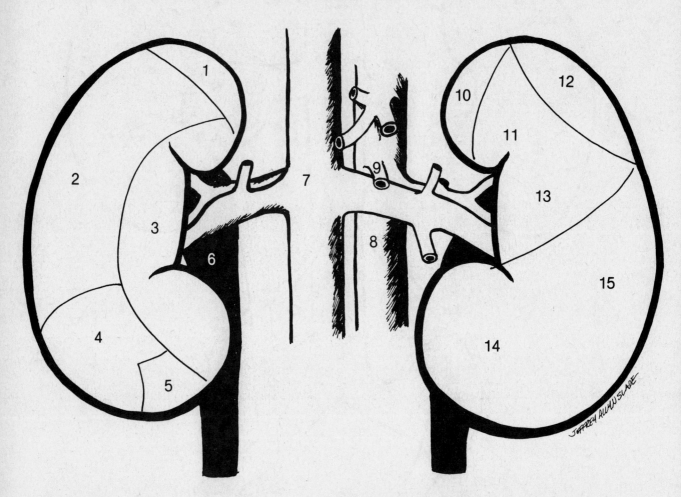

¹Right adrenal gland
²Liver
³Duodenum
⁴Right colic flexure
⁵Small intestine
⁶Ureter
⁷Inferior vena cava
⁸Aorta
⁹Superior mesenteric artery

¹⁰Left adrenal gland
¹¹Stomach
¹²Spleen
¹³Pancreas
¹⁴Jejunum
¹⁵Descending colon

Fig. 173 CORONAL SECTION OF THE KIDNEYS AS VIEWED FROM POSTERIOR

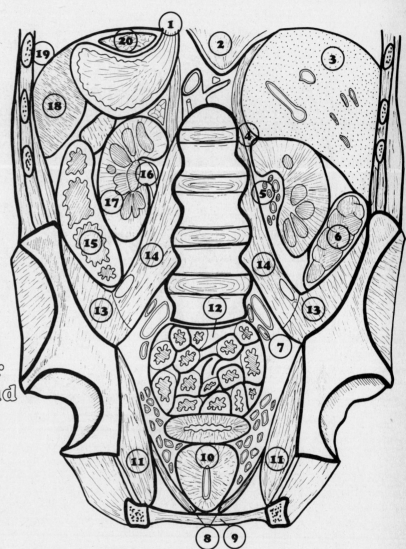

1 Cardiac orifice of the stomach
2 Diaphragm
3 Right lobe of the liver
4 Right suprarenal gland
5 Renal sinus
6 Ascending colon
7 Iliac artery and vein
8 Levator ani muscle
9 Transverse perineal muscle
10 Prostate
11 Obturator internus muscle
12 Ileum
13 Iliacus muscle
14 Psoas major muscle
15 Descending colon
16 Renal pelvis
17 Renal capsule
18 Spleen
19 Costodiaphragmatic recess
20 Left lobe of the liver

Fig. 174 SERIAL CROSS SECTION OF THE KIDNEYS, LEVEL 1

SERIAL CROSS SECTIONS OF
THE KIDNEY (Figs. 174
Through 178)

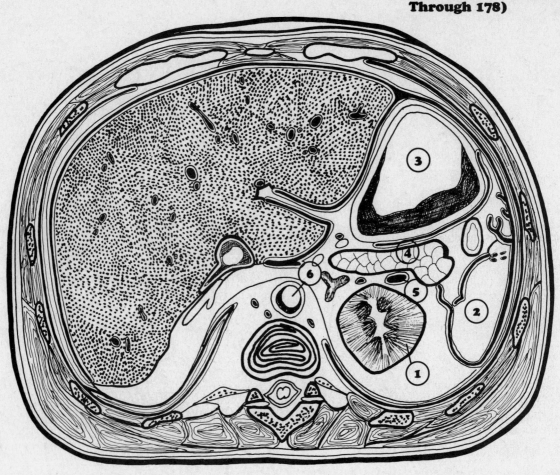

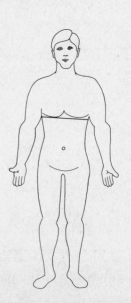

¹Left kidney
²Spleen
³Stomach
⁴Pancreas
⁵Splenic vein
⁶Aorta

Fig. 175 SERIAL CROSS SECTION OF THE KIDNEYS, LEVEL 2

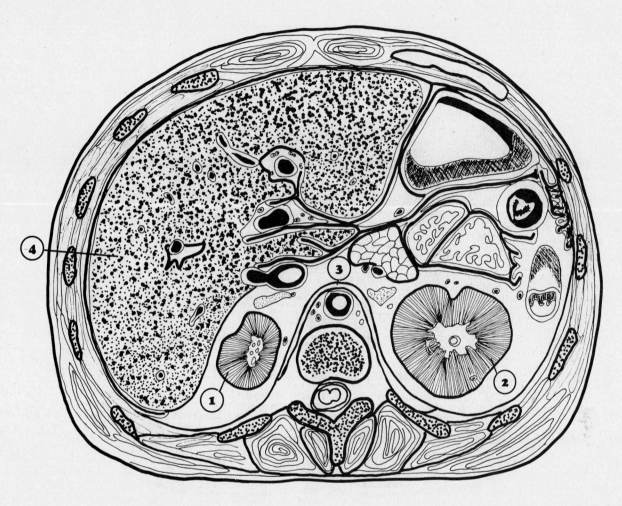

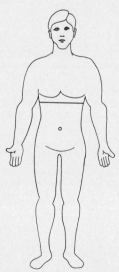

¹Right kidney
²Left kidney
³Crus of the diaphragm
⁴Right lobe of the liver

Fig. 176 SERIAL CROSS SECTION OF THE KIDNEYS, LEVEL 3

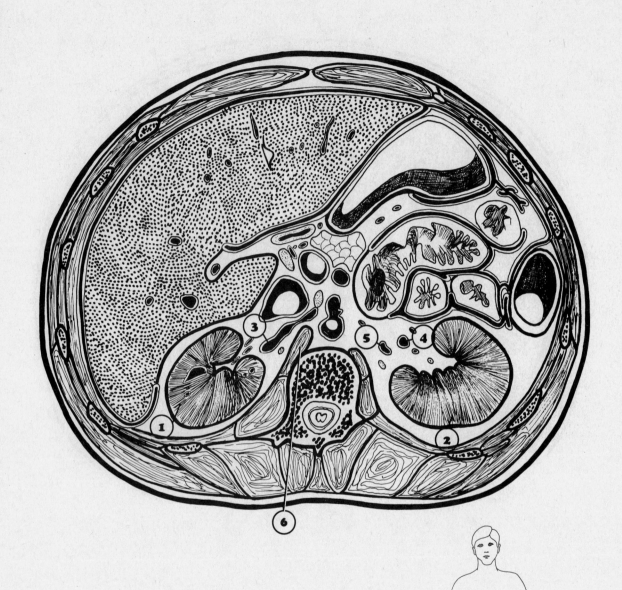

¹Right kidney
²Left kidney
³Right renal artery
⁴Left renal vein
⁵Left renal artery
⁶Crus of the diaphragm

Fig. 177 SERIAL CROSS SECTION OF THE KIDNEYS, LEVEL 4

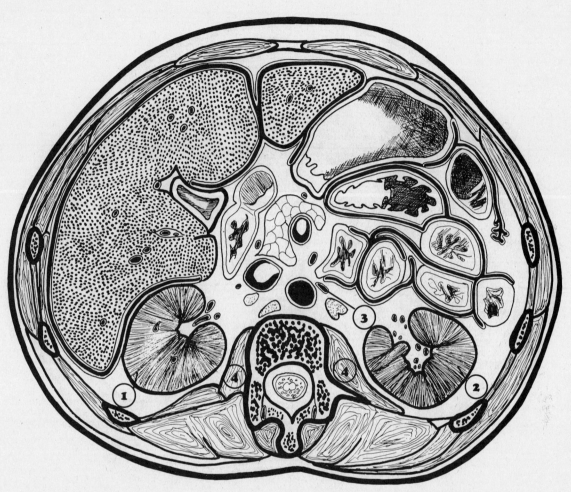

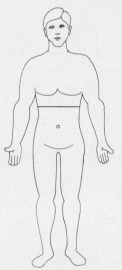

¹Right kidney
²Left kidney
³Left renal vein
⁴Psoas muscle

Fig. 178 SERIAL CROSS SECTION OF THE KIDNEYS, LEVEL 5

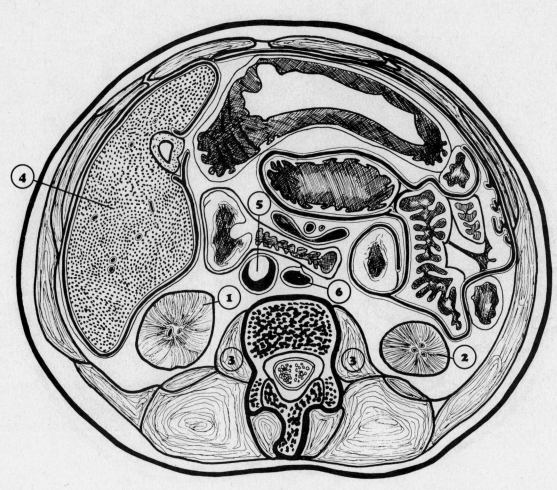

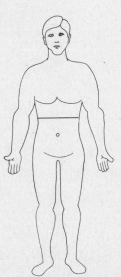

¹Right kidney
²Left kidney
³Psoas muscle
⁴Right lobe of the liver
⁵Inferior vena cava
⁶Aorta

Fig. 179 ABDOMINAL SAGITTAL SECTION, LEVEL 3

SERIAL SAGITTAL SECTIONS OF THE KIDNEY (Figs. 179 Through 183)

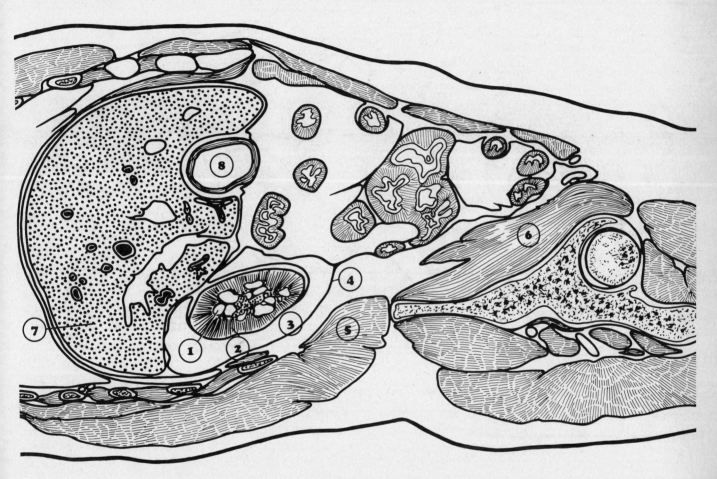

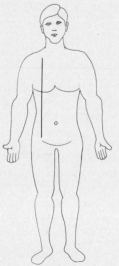

1 Right renal pyramid
2 Renal cortex
3 Perirenal fat
4 Perirenal fascia
5 Quadratus lumborum muscle
6 Iliacus muscle
7 Right lobe of the liver
8 Gallbladder

Fig. 180 ABDOMINAL SAGITTAL SECTION, LEVEL 4

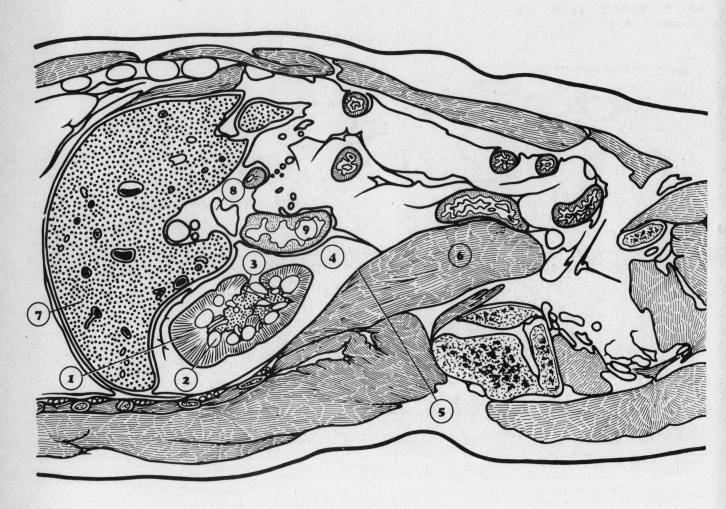

¹Right kidney
²Renal pyramid
³Renal sinus
⁴Perirenal fat
⁵Perirenal fascia
⁶Psoas major muscle
⁷Right lobe of liver
⁸Gallbladder neck
⁹Descending part of
   duodenum

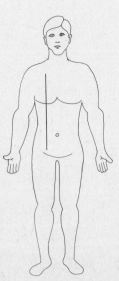

Fig. 181 ABDOMINAL SAGITTAL SECTION, LEVEL 5

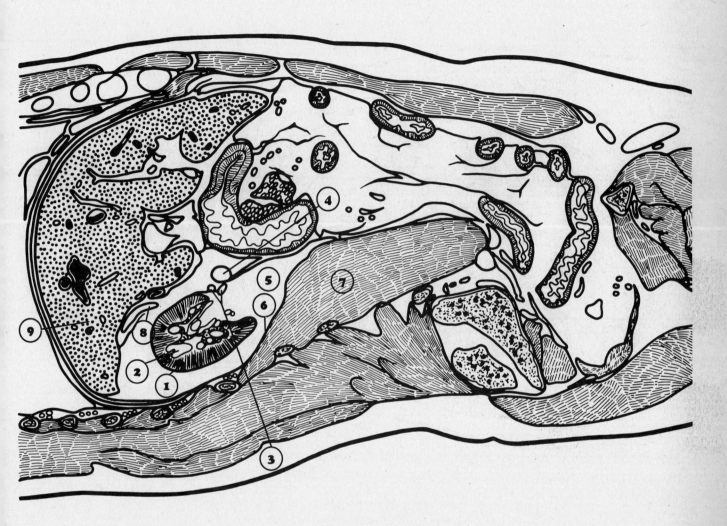

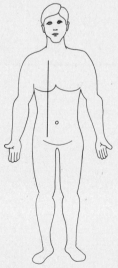

1 Right kidney
2 Renal pyramid
3 Right renal artery
4 Right renal vein
5 Perirenal fat
6 Perirenal fascia
7 Psoas major muscle
8 Right suprarenal gland
9 Right lobe of the liver

Fig. 182 ABDOMINAL SAGITTAL SECTION, LEVEL 6

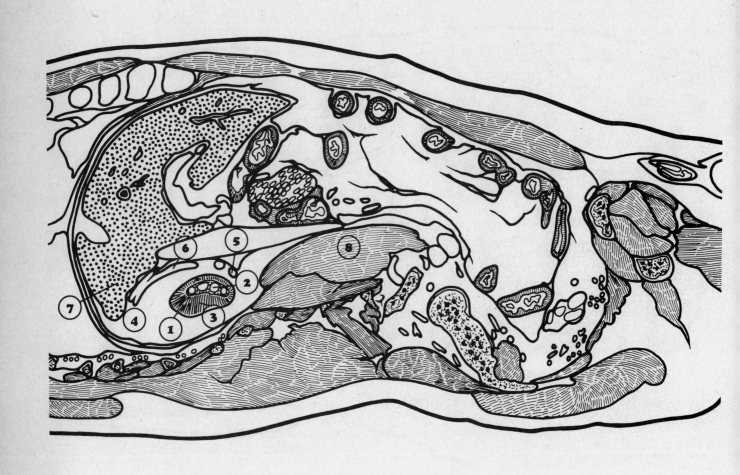

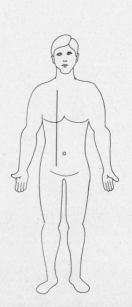

[1] Right kidney
[2] Renal medulla
[3] Renal cortex
[4] Perirenal fat
[5] Renal artery
[6] Right suprarenal gland
[7] Right lobe of the liver
[8] Psoas major muscle

Fig. 183 ABDOMINAL SAGITTAL SECTION, LEVEL 12

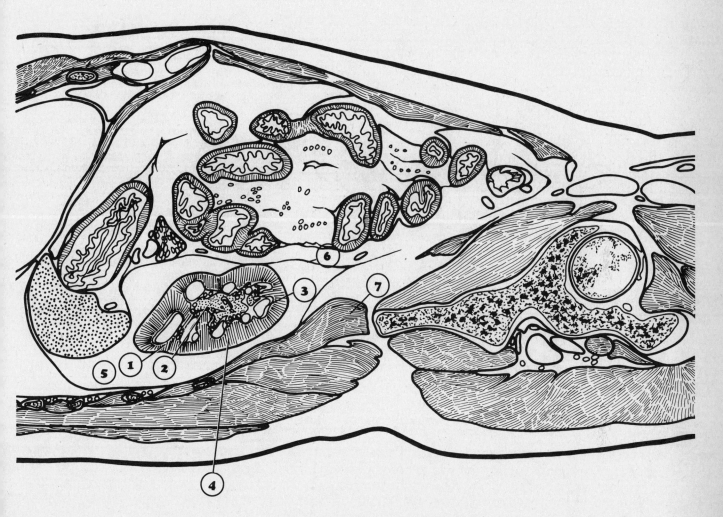

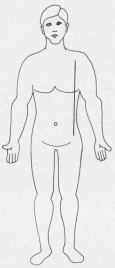

¹Left kidney
²Renal sinus
³Renal medulla
⁴Renal cortex
⁵Perirenal fat
⁶Perirenal fascia
⁷Quadratus lumborum
  muscle

Fig. 184 ADRENAL GLANDS

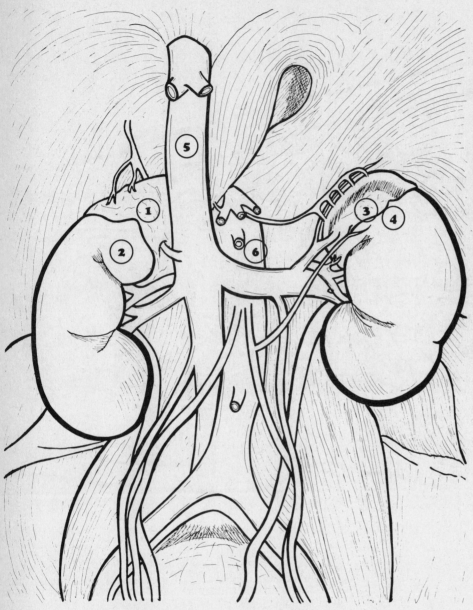

ADRENAL GLANDS

The adrenal glands are retroperitoneal organs that lie on the upper pole of each kidney (Fig. 184). They are surrounded by perinephric fascia and are separated from the kidneys by perinephric fat. Each gland has a cortex and a medulla.

The right adrenal gland is triangular or pyramidal and caps the upper pole of the right kidney. It lies posterior to the right lobe of the liver, extends medially behind the inferior vena cava, and rests posteriorly on the diaphragm.

The left adrenal gland is semilunar and extends along the medial border of the left kidney (from the upper pole to the hilum). It lies posterior to the pancreas, the lesser sac, and the stomach, and rests posteriorly on the diaphragm.

There are three arteries supplying each gland: the suprarenal branch of the inferior phrenic artery, the suprarenal branch of the aorta, and the suprarenal branch of the renal artery (Fig. 185). A single vein arises from the hilum of each gland and drains into the inferior vena cava on the right and into the renal vein on the left.

¹Right adrenal gland
²Upper pole of the right
  kidney
³Left adrenal gland
⁴Upper pole of the left
  kidney
⁵Inferior vena cava
⁶Aorta

Fig. 185 ARTERIAL SUPPLY TO THE ADRENAL GLANDS

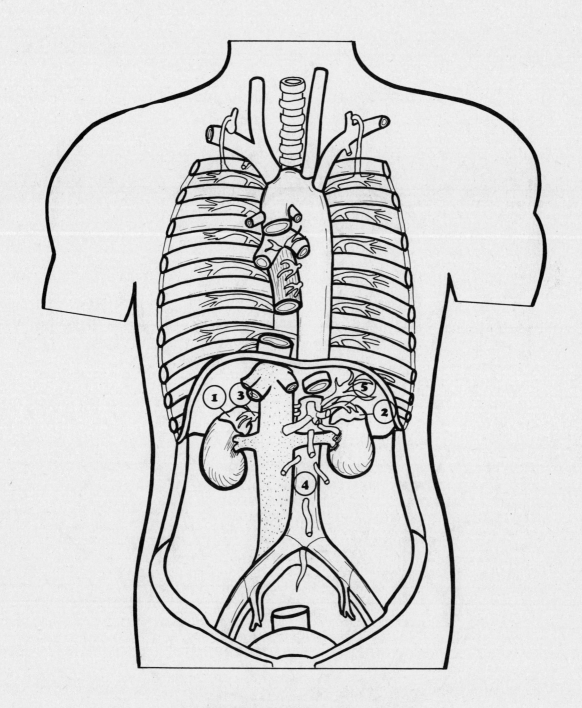

[1] Left adrenal gland
[2] Right adrenal gland
[3] Suprarenal arteries
[4] Abdominal aorta

Fig. 186 CORONAL SECTION OF THE ADRENAL GLAND AS VIEWED FROM POSTERIOR

CORONAL SECTION OF
THE ADRENAL GLAND
(Fig. 186)

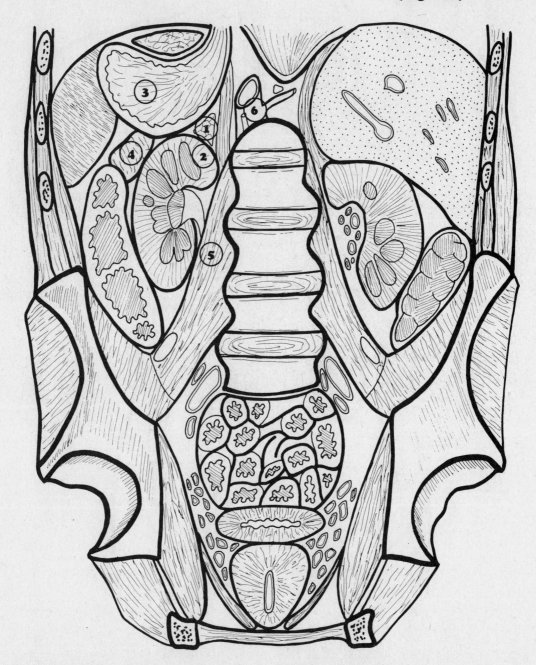

¹Left adrenal gland   ⁴Tail of the pancreas
²Left kidney   ⁵Psoas muscle
³Stomach   ⁶Aorta

198

Fig. 187 SERIAL CROSS SECTION OF
THE ADRENAL GLANDS, LEVEL 2

**SERIAL CROSS SECTIONS OF
THE ADRENAL GLANDS
(Figs. 187 and 188)**

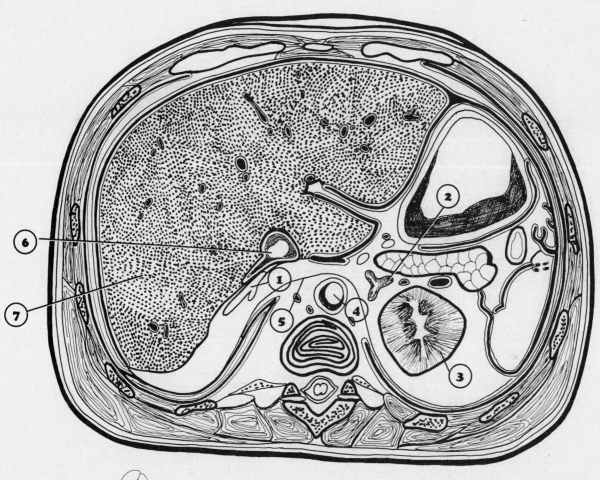

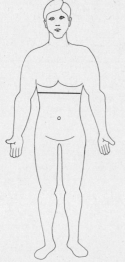

¹Right adrenal gland
²Left adrenal gland
³Left kidney
⁴Aorta
⁵Diaphragm
⁶Inferior vena cava
⁷Right lobe of the liver

199

Fig. 188 SERIAL CROSS SECTION OF THE ADRENAL GLANDS, LEVEL 3

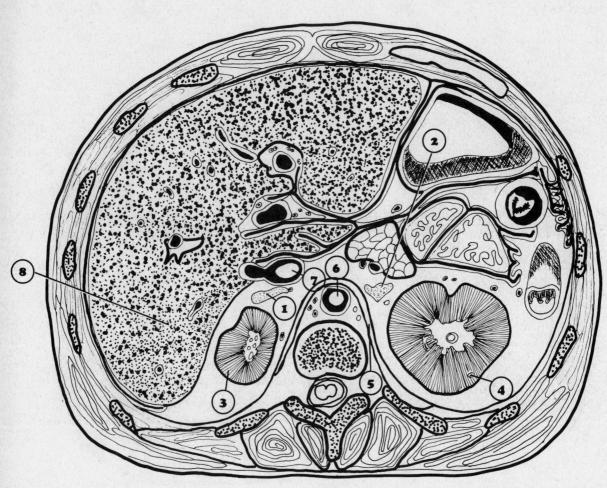

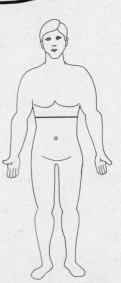

¹Right adrenal gland
²Left adrenal gland
³Right kidney
⁴Left kidney
⁵Crus of the diaphragm
⁶Aorta
⁷Inferior vena cava
⁸Right lobe of the liver

Fig. 189 ABDOMINAL SAGITTAL SECTION, LEVEL 5

**SERIAL SAGITTAL SECTIONS
OF THE ADRENAL GLANDS
(Figs. 189 Through 192)**

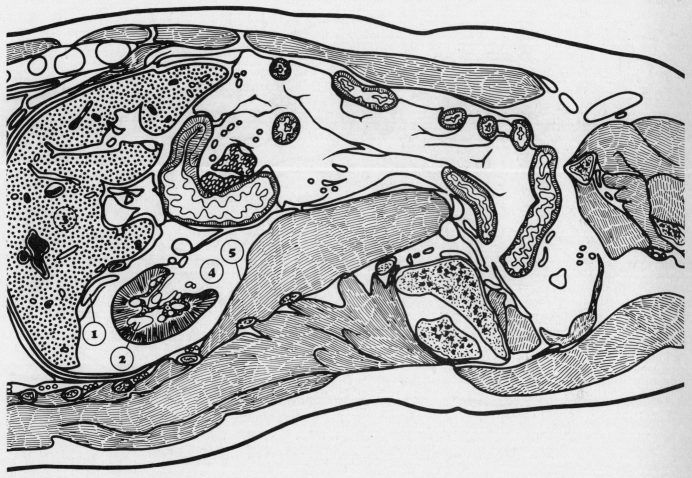

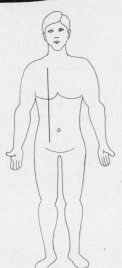

[1]Right suprarenal gland
[2]Right kidney
[3]Right lobe of the liver
[4]Perirenal fat
[5]Perirenal fascia

Fig. 190 ABDOMINAL SAGITTAL SECTION, LEVEL 6

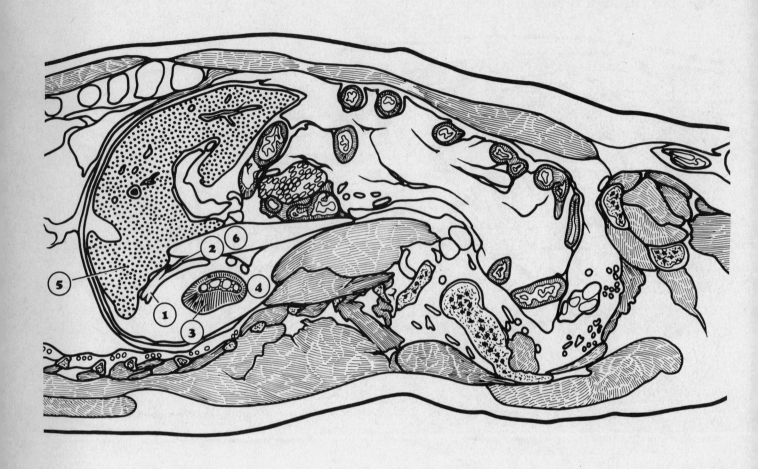

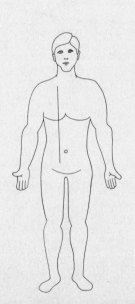

¹Right suprarenal gland
²Right suprarenal vein
³Right kidney
⁴Perirenal fat
⁵Right lobe of the liver
⁶Inferior vena cava

Fig. 191 ABDOMINAL SAGITTAL SECTION, LEVEL 7

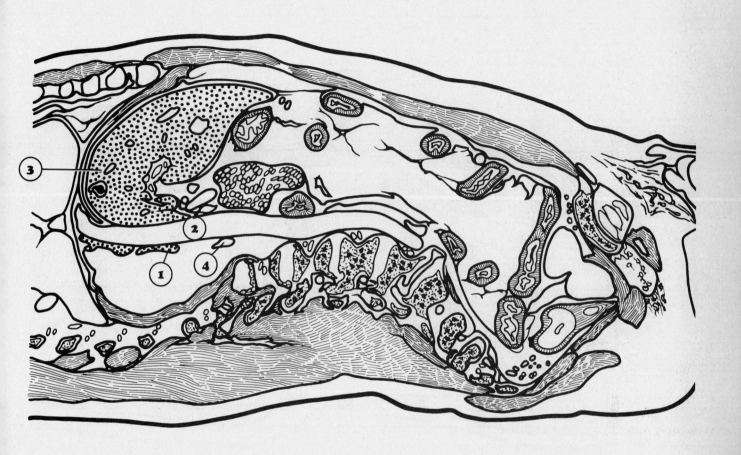

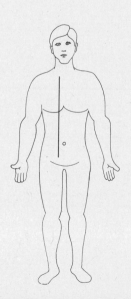

[1] Right suprarenal gland
[2] Inferior vena cava
[3] Left lobe of the liver
[4] Right renal artery

Fig. 192 ABDOMINAL SAGITTAL SECTION, LEVEL 12

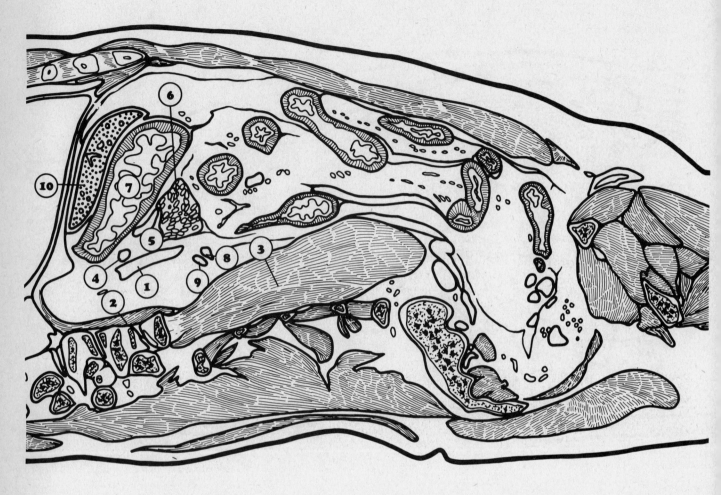

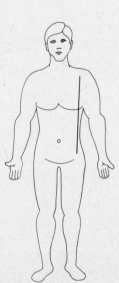

1 Left suprarenal gland
2 Crus of the diaphragm
3 Psoas major muscle
4 Splenic artery
5 Splenic vein
6 Pancreas
7 Body of the stomach
8 Left renal vein
9 Left renal artery
10 Left lobe of the liver

Review of the Abdomen

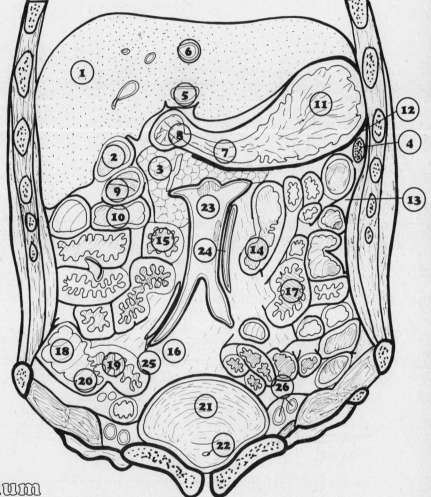

1 Liver
2 Gallbladder
3 Pancreas
4 Spleen
5 Portal vein
6 Hepatic vein
7 Pylorus
8 Pyloric sphincter
9 Transverse colon
10 Intestine
11 Stomach
12 Omental bursa
13 Greater omentum
14 Ascending duodenum
15 Inferior duodenum
16 Mesentery
17 Jejunum
18 Ascending colon
19 Ileum
20 Cecum
21 Bladder
22 Urethral ostium
23 Superior mesenteric artery
24 Superior mesenteric vein
25 Ileocolic artery and vein
26 External iliac artery and vein

205

Fig. 194 ABDOMINAL CROSS SECTION, LEVEL 1

ABDOMEN, LEVEL 1
(Fig. 194)

This cross section is made at the level of the tenth intervertebral disc. The lower portion of the pericardial sac is seen in this section. The splenic artery enters the spleen, and the splenic vein emerges from the splenic hilum. The abdominal portion of the esophagus lies to the left of the midline and opens into the stomach through the cardiac orifice. The liver extends to the left mammillary line. The coronary ligament is shown. The falciform ligament extends into the section above this. The upper border of the tail of the pancreas and the body of this structure are shown. The spleen is seen to lie alongside the ninth rib. The upper pole of the left kidney is seen posterior to the spleen.

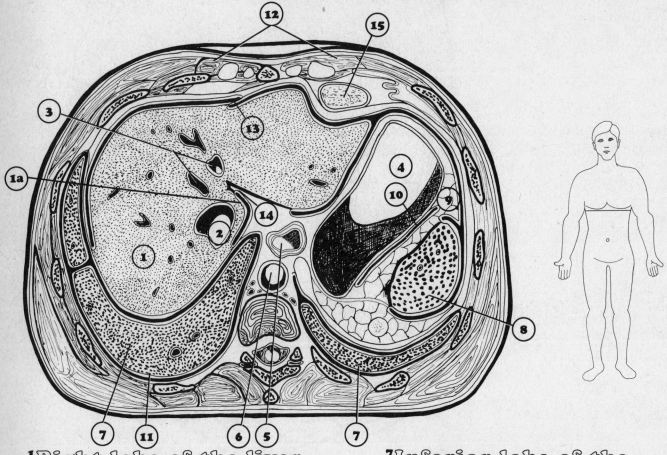

¹**Right lobe of the liver**
¹ᵃ**Caudate lobe**
²**Inferior vena cava**
³**Hepatic veins**
⁴**Stomach**
⁵**Esophagus**
⁶**Abdominal aorta**
⁷**Inferior lobe of the lung**
⁸**Spleen**
⁹**Gastrosplenic ligament**
¹⁰**Omental bursa**
¹¹**Pleural sac**
¹²**Rectus abdominis muscle**
¹³**Falciform ligament**
¹⁴**Ligamentum venosum**
¹⁵**Pericardial sac**

Fig. 195 ABDOMINAL CROSS SECTION, LEVEL 2

ABDOMEN, LEVEL 2
(Fig. 195)

This section is taken at the level of the eleventh thoracic disc and the superior portion of the twelfth thoracic vertebra. The hepatic vein is shown to enter the inferior vena cava. The renal artery and the vein of the left kidney are shown. The left branch of the portal vein is seen to arch upward to enter the left lobe of the liver. The upper part of the stomach is shown with the hepatogastric and gastrocolic ligaments. The lesser omental cavity is behind the stomach. The upper border of the splenic flexure of the colon is seen. The falciform and coronary ligaments of the liver can be seen. The caudate lobe of the liver is seen in this section and in Level 1. The tail and body of the pancreas are seen. The spleen is shown along the left lateral border. The adrenal glands are shown lateral to the crus of the diaphragm.

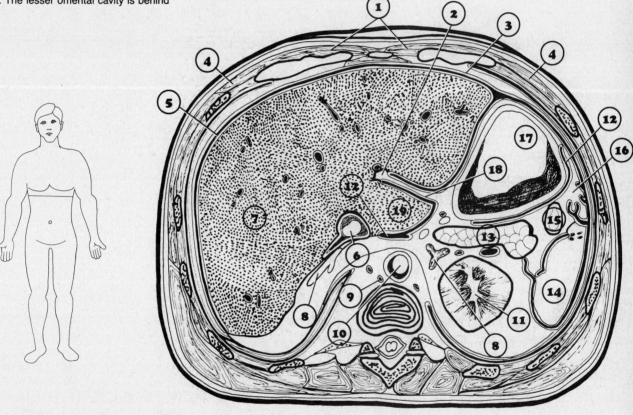

¹Rectus abdominis muscle

²Ligamentum venosum

³Diaphragm

⁴External oblique muscle

⁵Peritoneal cavity

⁶Inferior vena cava

⁷Right lobe of the liver

⁸Suprarenal glands

⁹Azygos vein

¹⁰Aorta

¹¹Kidney

¹²Omental bursa

¹³Pancreas

¹⁴Spleen

¹⁵Colic flexure

¹⁶Gastric ligament

¹⁷Stomach

¹⁸Hepatogastric ligament

¹⁹Caudate lobe of the liver

Fig. 196 ABDOMINAL CROSS SECTION, LEVEL 3

ABDOMEN, LEVEL 3
(Fig. 196)

This section is taken at the level of the twelfth thoracic vertebra, slightly above the intervertebral disc. The celiac axis (not shown) arises in the middle of this section from the anterior abdominal aorta. The right renal artery originates in this section. Again, one of the hepatic veins is shown to enter the inferior vena cava. The section cuts through the mid portion of the greater curvature of the stomach and includes part of the pylorus of the stomach. A small portion of the superior portion of the duo-denum is found in the lower part of this section. The ligament of Treitz is shown. The transverse and descending colon are shown below the splenic flexure. (The descending colon is a retroperitoneal structure.) The transverse mesocolon is shown. The falciform ligament, right triangular ligament, and gastro-hepatic omentum are shown. The caudate lobe of the liver is well seen. The body of the pancreas, both kidneys, and the lower portions of the adrenal glands are shown.

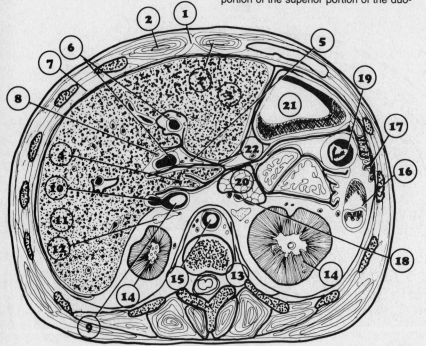

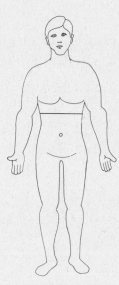

¹Linea alba
²Rectus abdominis muscle
³Left lobe of the liver
⁴Caudate lobe of the liver
⁵Hepatic artery
⁶Portal vein
⁷Diaphragm
⁸Hepatic duct
⁹Inferior vena cava
¹⁰Hepatic vein

¹¹Right lobe of the liver
¹²Suprarenal gland
¹³Crus of the diaphragm
¹⁴Kidney
¹⁵Aorta
¹⁶Descending colon
¹⁷Peritoneal cavity
¹⁸Splenic vein
¹⁹Transverse colon
²⁰Pancreas
²¹Stomach
²²Omental bursa

Fig. 197 ABDOMINAL CROSS SECTION, LEVEL 4

ABDOMEN, LEVEL 4
(Fig. 197)

This section is taken at the level of the first lumbar vertebra. The psoas major muscle is seen. The crura of the diaphragm are shown on each side of the vertebra. The right renal artery is shown. The left renal artery arises from the lateral wall of the aorta. Both renal veins enter the inferior vena cava. The portal vein is seen to be formed by the union of the splenic vein and the superior mesenteric vein. The lower portion of the stomach and the py-

loric orifice are seen, as is the superior portion of the duodenum. The duodenojejunal flexure and descending and transverse colon are shown. The greater omentum is very prominent. The small, nonperitoneal area of the liver is shown anterior to the right kidney. The round ligament of the liver and the umbilical fissure, which separates the right and left lobes of the liver, are seen. The neck of the gallbladder (not shown) is found just inferior to

this section, between the quadrate and caudate lobes of the liver. The cystic duct is cut in two places. The hepatic duct lies just anterior to the cystic duct. The cystic and hepatic ducts unite in the lower part of the section to form the common bile duct. The pancreatic duct is found within the pancreas at this level. Both kidneys are seen just lateral to the psoas muscles.

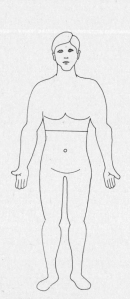

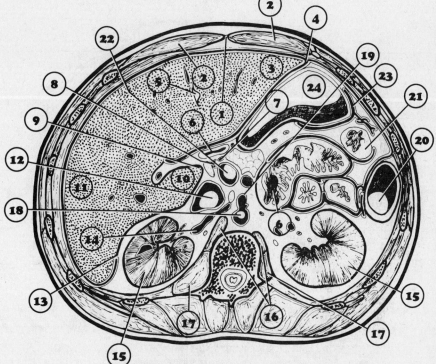

¹Linea alba
²Rectus abdominis muscle
³Left lobe of the liver
⁴Peritoneal cavity
⁵Ligamentum teres
⁶Duodenum
⁷Gastroduodenal artery
⁸Hepatic duct
⁹Epiploic foramen (foramen of Winslow)
¹⁰Caudate lobe of the liver
¹¹Right lobe of the liver

¹²Inferior vena cava
¹³Hepatorenal ligament
¹⁴Renal artery
¹⁵Kidney
¹⁶Crus of the diaphragm
¹⁷Psoas major muscle
¹⁸Aorta
¹⁹Superior mesenteric artery
²⁰Descending colon
²¹Transverse colon
²²Splenic vein
²³Omental bursa
²⁴Stomach

Fig. 198 ABDOMINAL CROSS SECTION, LEVEL 5

ABDOMEN, LEVEL 5
(Fig. 198)

This section is taken at the level of the second lumbar vertebra. The superior pancreaticoduodenal artery originates in Level 4 and shows some of its branches on this section. The lower portion of the stomach is found in this section, and the hepatic flexure of the colon is seen. The lobes of the liver are separated by the round ligament. The left lobe of the liver ends at this level. The head and neck of the pancreas drape around the superior mesenteric vein. Both kidneys and the psoas muscles are shown.

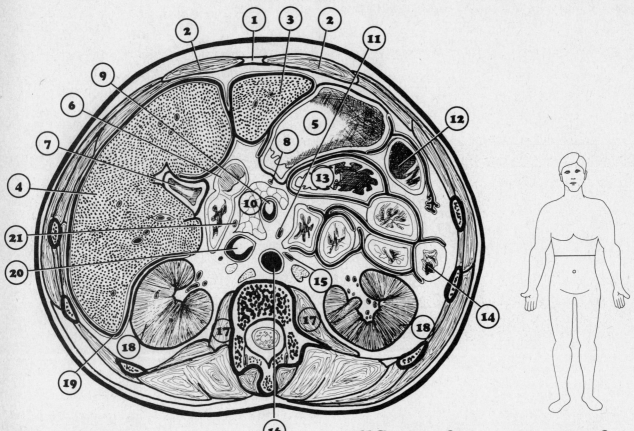

1 Linea alba
2 Rectus abdominis muscle
3 Left lobe of the liver
4 Right lobe of the liver
5 Stomach
6 Duodenum
7 Gallbladder
8 Gastroduodenal artery
9 Superior mesenteric vein
10 Pancreas
11 Superior mesenteric artery
12 Transverse colon
13 Jejunum
14 Descending colon
15 Left renal vein
16 Aorta
17 Psoas major muscle
18 Kidney
19 Peritoneal cavity
20 Inferior vena cava
21 Common bile duct

Fig. 199 ABDOMINAL CROSS SECTION, LEVEL 6

ABDOMEN, LEVEL 6
(Fig. 199)

This section is taken at the level of the third lumbar vertebra. The inferior mesenteric artery originates from the abdominal aorta at this level. The greater omentum is shown mostly on the left side of the abdomen. The descending and ascending portions of the duodenum, which lie between the aorta and the superior mesenteric artery and vein, are shown. The fundus of the gallbladder lies in the lower portion of this section. The lower poles of both kidneys lie lateral to the psoas muscles.

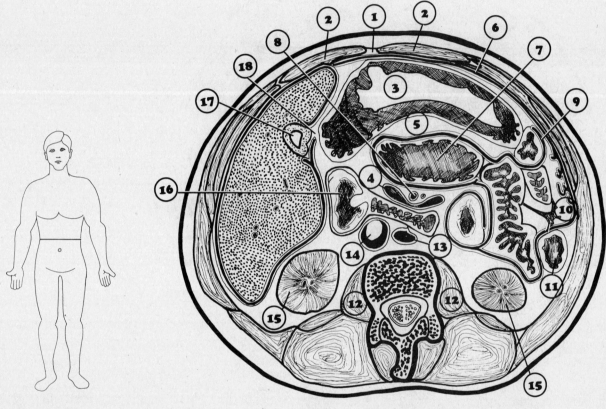

1 Linea alba
2 Rectus abdominis muscle
3 Transverse colon
4 Superior mesenteric vein
5 Transverse mesocolon
6 Parietal peritoneum
7 Jejunum
8 Superior mesenteric artery
9 Peritoneal cavity
10 Greater omentum
11 Descending colon
12 Psoas major muscle
13 Aorta
14 Inferior vena cava
15 Kidney
16 Duodenum
17 Gallbladder
18 Hepatocolic ligament

211

Fig. 200 ABDOMINAL CROSS SECTION, LEVEL 7

This section is taken through the third lumbar disc. The lower portion of the duodenum is shown. The section passes through many loops of jejunum and ileum. The lower margin of the right lobe of the liver is shown along the right lateral border.

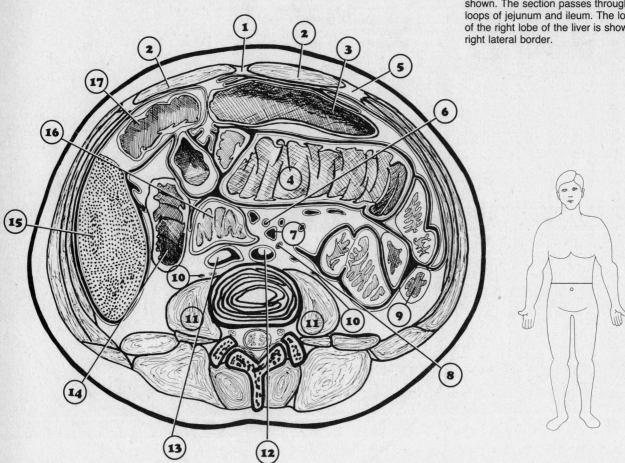

¹Linea alba
²Rectus abdominis muscle
³Transverse colon
⁴Jejunum
⁵Linea semilunaris
⁶Superior mesenteric artery

⁷Superior mesenteric vein
⁸Inferior mesenteric artery
⁹Descending colon
¹⁰Ureter
¹¹Psoas major muscle
¹²Aorta
¹³Inferior vena cava
¹⁴Ascending colon
¹⁵Right lobe of the liver
¹⁶Duodenum
¹⁷Ileum

Fig. 201 ABDOMINAL CROSS SECTION, LEVEL 8

ABDOMEN, LEVEL 8 (Fig. 201)

This section is taken through the lower portion of the fourth lumbar vertebra. The aorta bifurcates into the common iliac arteries in this section, and coils of small intestine are seen throughout. The coils on the left side are through the jejunal portion; those on the right side are through the ileal portion. The ascending and descending colons are shown. The greater omentum is still prominent on the left side.

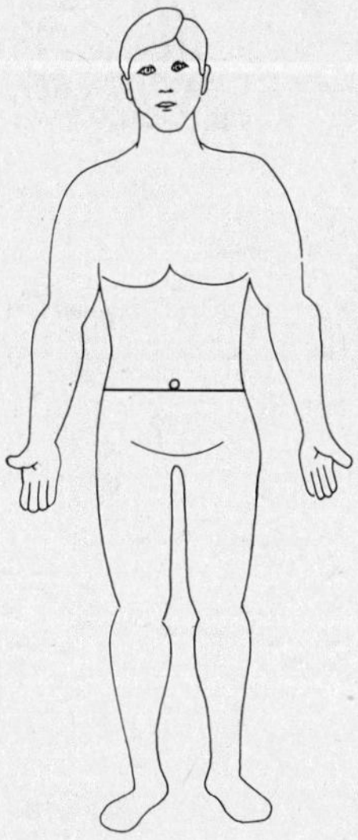

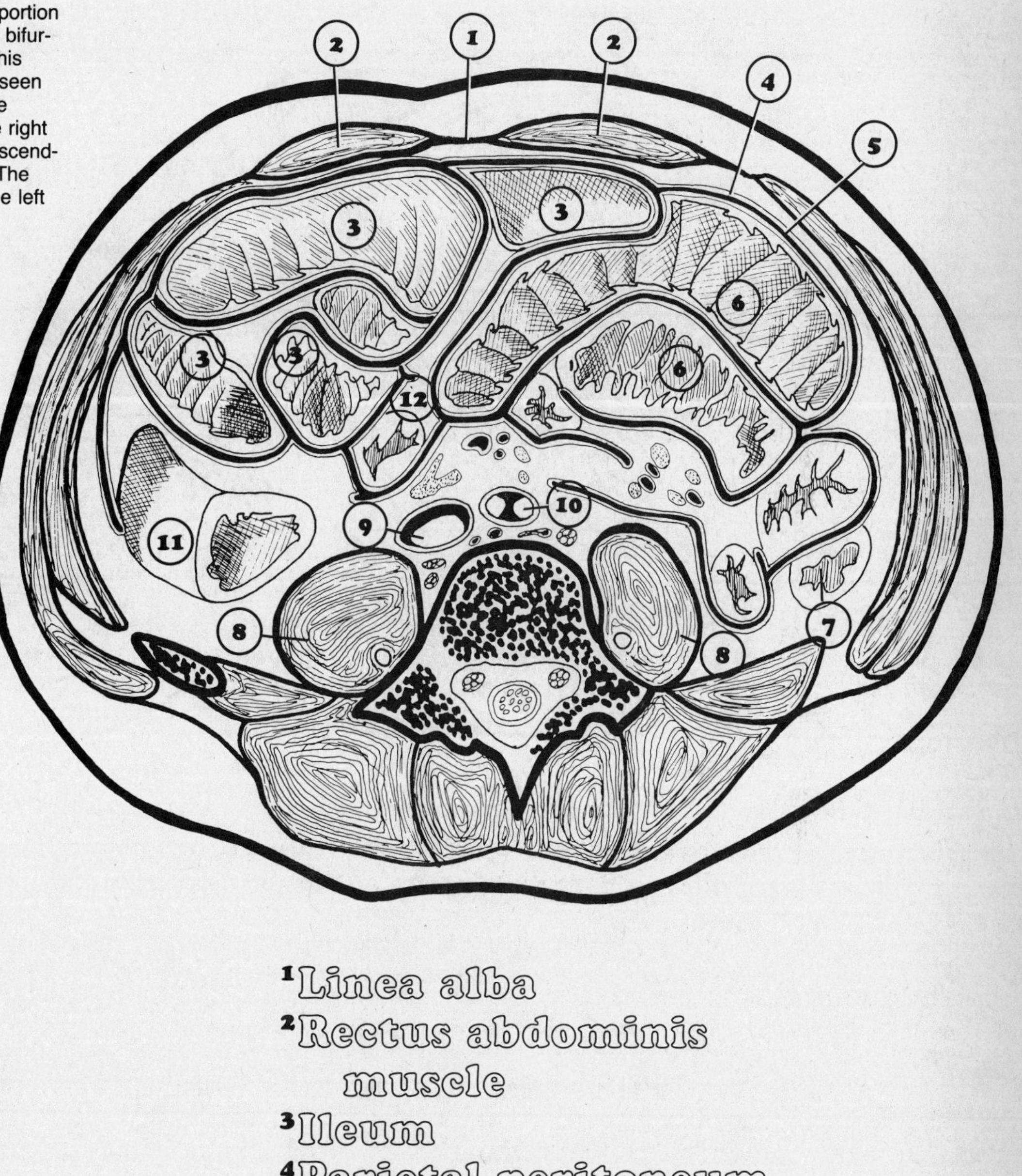

1 Linea alba
2 Rectus abdominis muscle
3 Ileum
4 Parietal peritoneum
5 Peritoneal cavity
6 Jejunum
7 Descending colon
8 Psoas muscle
9 Inferior vena cava
10 Aortic bifurcation
11 Ascending colon
12 Mesentery

213

Fig. 202 ABDOMINAL SAGITTAL SECTION, LEVEL 1

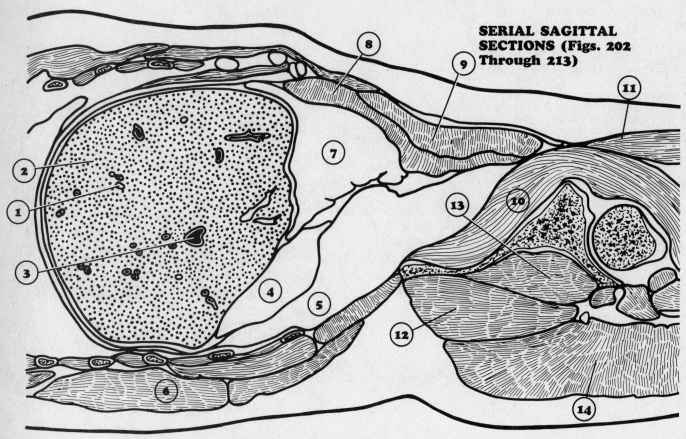

SERIAL SAGITTAL
SECTIONS (Figs. 202
Through 213)

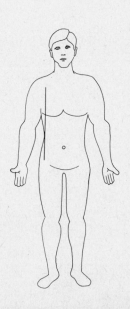

1 Portal vein
2 Right lobe of the liver
3 Hepatic vein
4 Perirenal fat
5 Retroperitoneal fat
6 Latissimus dorsi muscle
7 Omentum
8 Internal oblique muscle
9 External oblique
   muscle
10 Iliacus muscle
11 Psoas major muscle
12 Gluteus medius muscle
13 Gluteus minimus
    muscle
14 Gluteus maximus
    muscle

Fig. 203 ABDOMINAL SAGITTAL SECTION, LEVEL 2

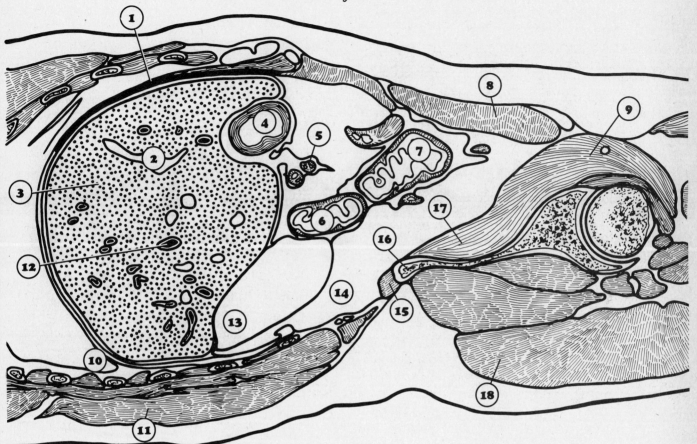

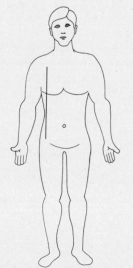

1 Diaphragm
2 Portal vein
3 Liver
4 Gallbladder
5 Hepatic flexure
6 Ascending colon
7 Cecum
8 Internal oblique muscle
9 Psoas major muscle
10 Costodiaphragmatic
   recess
11 Latissimus dorsi muscle
12 Hepatic vein
13 Perirenal fat
14 Retroperitoneal fat
15 Quadratus lumborum
   muscle

16 Ilium
17 Iliacus muscle
18 Gluteus maximus
   muscle

Fig. 204 ABDOMINAL SAGITTAL SECTION, LEVEL 3

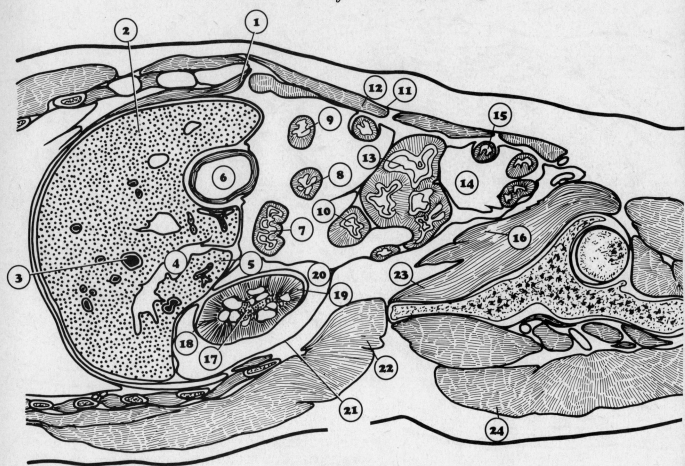

¹Diaphragm
²Liver
³Hepatic vein
⁴Portal vein
⁵Caudate lobe of the liver
⁶Gallbladder
⁷Hepatic flexure
⁸Transverse colon
⁹Small bowel
¹⁰Ascending colon
¹¹Rectus sheath
¹²Rectus abdominis muscle

¹³Cecum
¹⁴Mesentery
¹⁵Small bowel
¹⁶Psoas major muscle
¹⁷Renal medulla
¹⁸Right kidney
¹⁹Renal cortex
²⁰Perirenal fat
²¹Perirenal fascia
²²Quadratus lumborum muscle
²³Iliacus muscle
²⁴Gluteus maximus muscle

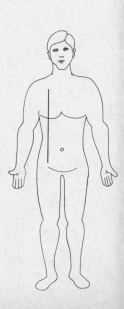

Fig. 205 ABDOMINAL SAGITTAL SECTION, LEVEL 4

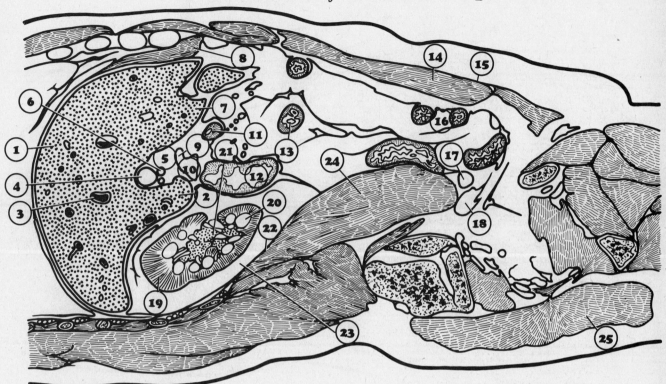

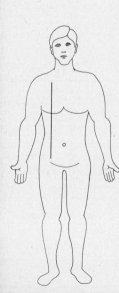

1 Liver
2 Caudate lobe of the liver
3 Hepatic vein
4 Portal vein
5 Porta hepatis
6 Hepatic artery
7 Quadrate lobe of the liver
8 Diaphragm
9 Neck of the gallbladder
10 Hartmann's pouch
11 Superior part of the duodenum
12 Descending part of the duodenum
13 Transverse colon

14 Rectus abdominis muscle
15 Anterior rectus sheath
16 Mesentery
17 Right external iliac artery
18 Right external iliac vein
19 Kidney
20 Renal pyramid
21 Renal sinus
22 Perirenal fascia
23 Perirenal fat
24 Psoas major muscle
25 Gluteus maximus muscle

Fig. 206 ABDOMINAL SAGITTAL SECTION, LEVEL 5

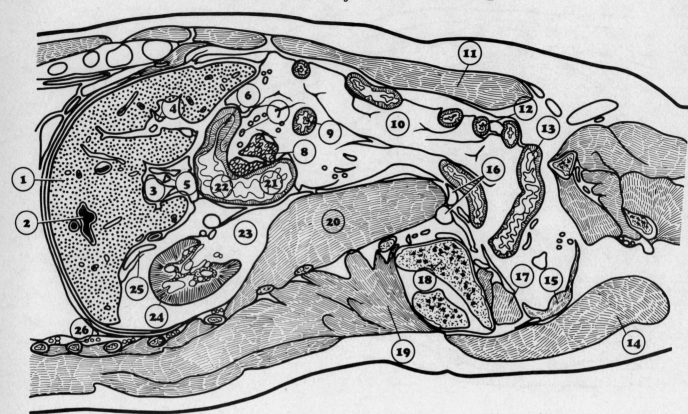

1. Right lobe of the liver
2. Hepatic vein
3. Portal vein
4. Left branch of the portal vein
5. Cystic duct
6. Pyloric sphincter
7. Gastroduodenal artery
8. Head of the pancreas
9. Transverse colon
10. Mesentery
11. Rectus abdominis muscle
12. Small bowel
13. Ileum
14. Gluteus maximus muscle
15. Levator ani muscle
16. Right external iliac artery
17. Piriformis muscle
18. Sacrum
19. Erector spinae muscle
20. Psoas major muscle
21. Descending duodenum
22. Superior duodenum
23. Perirenal fat
24. Right kidney
25. Right suprarenal gland
26. Costodiaphragmatic recess

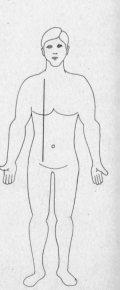

Fig. 207 ABDOMINAL SAGITTAL SECTION, LEVEL 6

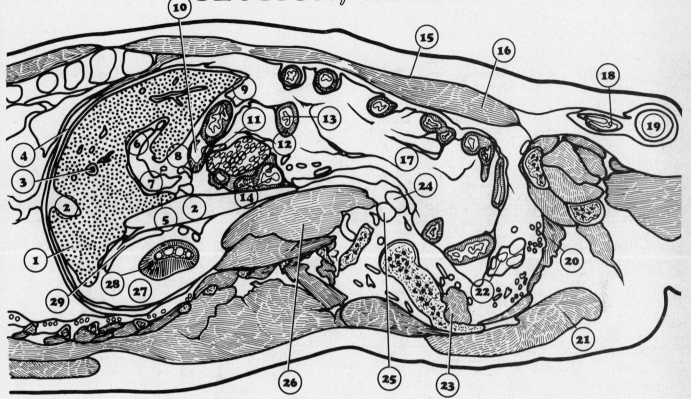

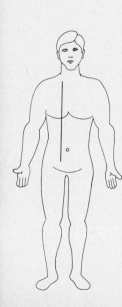

1 Right lobe of the liver
2 Inferior vena cava
3 Hepatic vein
4 Diaphragm
5 Caudate lobe of the liver
6 Left portal vein
7 Hepatic artery
8 Cystic duct
9 Pylorus
10 Descending part of the duodenum
11 Gastroduodenal artery
12 Head of the pancreas
13 Transverse colon
14 Superior part of the duodenum
15 Anterior rectus sheath

16 Rectus abdominis muscle
17 Mesenteric fat
18 Spermatic cord
19 Testis
20 Levator ani muscle
21 Gluteus maximus muscle
22 Seminal vesicles
23 Piriformis muscle
24 Right common iliac artery
25 Right common iliac vein
26 Psoas major muscle
27 Perirenal fat
28 Right kidney
29 Right suprarenal gland

Fig. 208 ABDOMINAL SAGITTAL SECTION, LEVEL 7

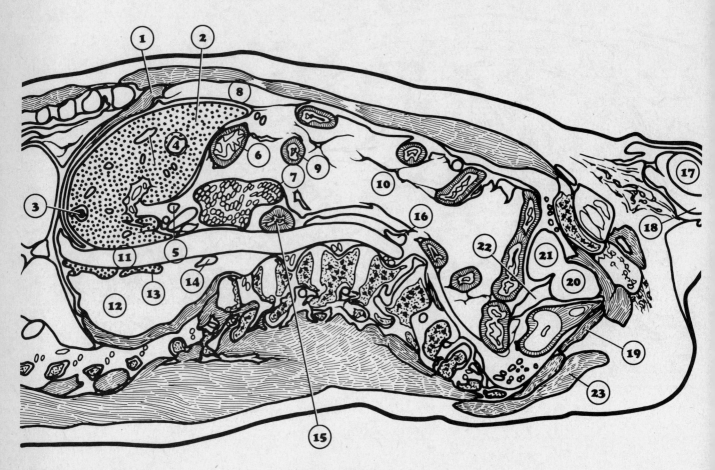

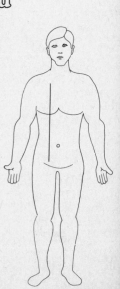

¹Diaphragm
²Left lobe of the liver
³Hepatic vein
⁴Portal vein
⁵Hepatic artery
⁶Pyloric antrum
⁷Head of the pancreas
⁸Falciform ligament
⁹Transverse colon
¹⁰Mesenteric fat

¹¹Inferior vena cava
¹²Perirenal fat
¹³Right suprarenal gland
¹⁴Right renal artery
¹⁵Horizontal part of the duodenum
¹⁶Right common iliac artery
¹⁷Testis
¹⁸Scrotum
¹⁹Levator ani muscle
²⁰Prostate
²¹Bladder
²²Seminal vesicles
²³Gluteus maximus muscle

Fig. 209 ABDOMINAL SAGITTAL SECTION, LEVEL 8

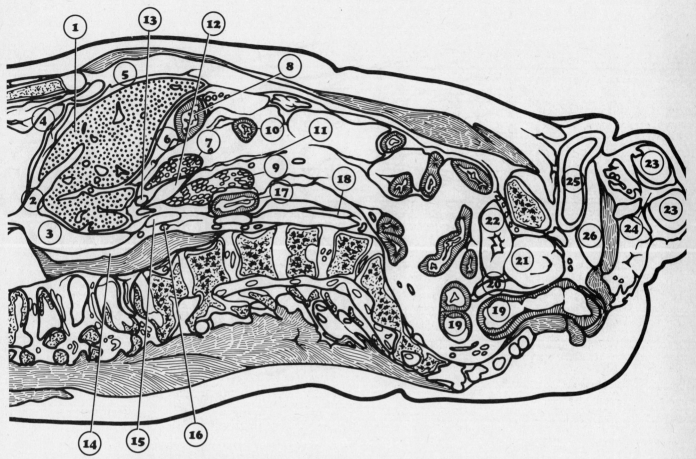

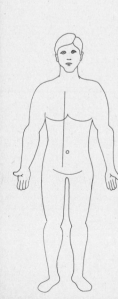

1 Left lobe of the liver
2 Hepatic vein
3 Inferior vena cava
4 Diaphragm
5 Falciform ligament
6 Lesser omentum
7 Pancreas
8 Pyloric antrum
9 Uncinate process of the pancreas
10 Transverse colon
11 Superior mesenteric vein
12 Portal vein
13 Hepatic artery
14 Crus of the diaphragm
15 Left renal vein
16 Right renal artery
17 Horizontal part of the duodenum
18 Right common iliac artery
19 Rectum
20 Seminal vesicles
21 Prostate
22 Bladder
23 Testis
24 Scrotum
25 Corpus cavernosum penis
26 Corpus spongiosum penis

Fig. 210 ABDOMINAL SAGITTAL SECTION, LEVEL 9

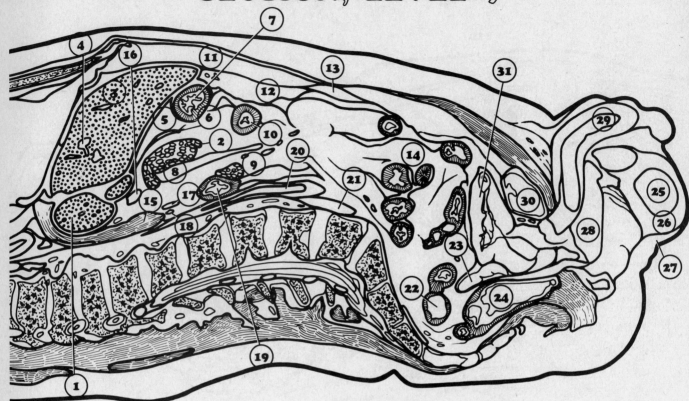

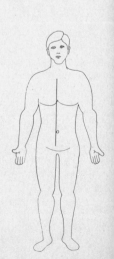

1. Caudate lobe of the liver
2. Body of the pancreas
3. Left lobe of the liver
4. Portal vein
5. Lesser omentum
6. Lesser sac
7. Pyloric antrum
8. Superior mesenteric vein
9. Uncinate process of the pancreas
10. Transverse colon
11. Falciform ligament
12. Greater omentum
13. Linea alba
14. Mesenteric fat
15. Crus of the diaphragm
16. Hepatic artery
17. Left renal vein
18. Right renal artery
19. Horizontal part of the duodenum
20. Aorta
21. Left common iliac vein
22. Rectum
23. Seminal vescioles
24. Rectum
25. Testis
26. Epididymis
27. Scrotum
28. Corpus spongiosum penis
29. Corpus cavernosum penis
30. Symphysis pubis
31. Bladder

Fig. 211 ABDOMINAL SAGITTAL SECTION, LEVEL 10

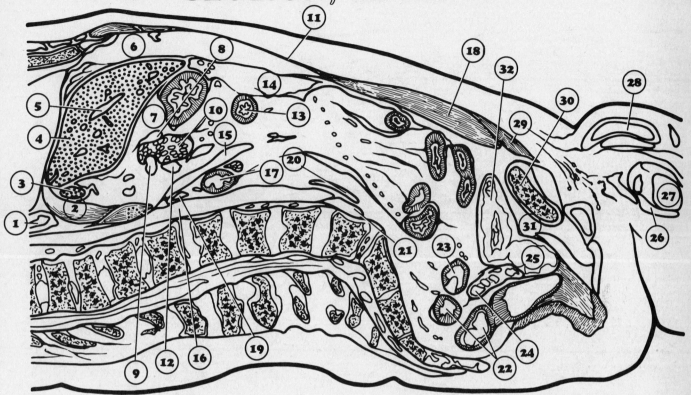

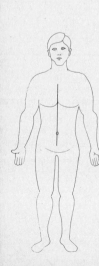

1 Esophagus
2 Crus of the diaphragm
3 Caudate lobe of the liver
4 Left lobe of the liver
5 Portal vein
6 Falciform ligament
7 Lesser omentum
8 Lesser sac
9 Splenic artery
10 Pancreas
11 Linea alba
12 Splenic vein
13 Transverse colon
14 Greater omentum
15 Superior mesenteric artery
16 Aorta
17 Horizontal part of the

duodenum
18 Rectus abdominis muscle
19 Left renal vein
20 Inferior mesenteric artery
21 Left common iliac vein
22 Rectum
23 Sigmoid colon
24 Seminal vesicles
25 Prostate
26 Head of the epididymis
27 Testis
28 Corpus cavernosum penis
29 Pyramidalis muscle
30 Symphysis pubis
31 Retropubic space
32 Bladder

Fig. 212 ABDOMINAL SAGITTAL SECTION, LEVEL 11

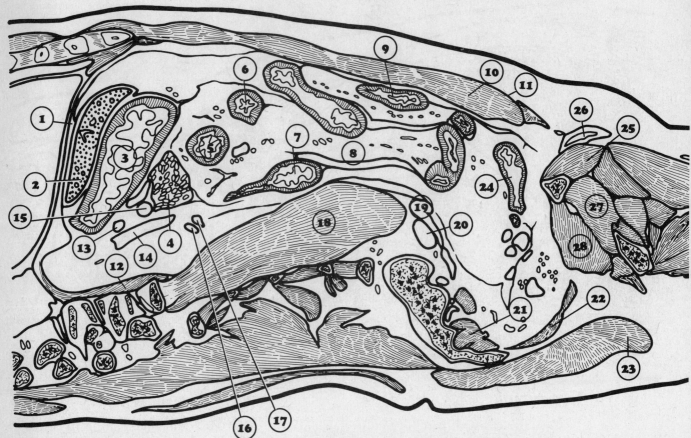

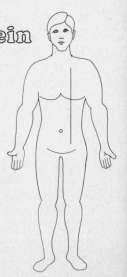

1 Diaphragm
2 Left lobe of the liver
3 Body of the stomach
4 Pancreas
5 Ascending part of the duodenum
6 Transverse colon
7 Jejunum
8 Mesentery
9 Small bowel
10 Rectus abdominis muscle
11 Rectus sheath
12 Crus of the diaphragm
13 Splenic artery
14 Left suprarenal gland
15 Splenic vein

16 Left renal artery
17 Left renal vein
18 Psoas major muscle
19 Left common iliac artery
20 Left common iliac vein
21 Piriformis muscle
22 Levator ani muscle
23 Gluteus maximus muscle
24 Sigmoid colon
25 Pectineus muscle
26 Spermatic cord
27 Obturator externus muscle
28 Obturator internus muscle

Fig. 213 ABDOMINAL SAGITTAL SECTION, LEVEL 12

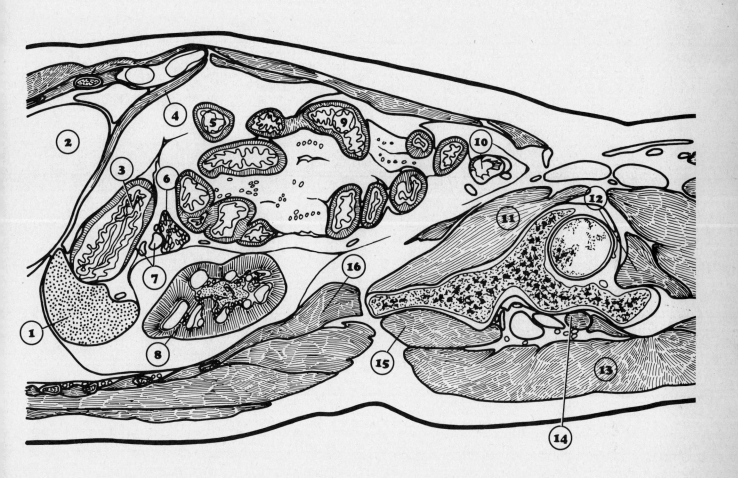

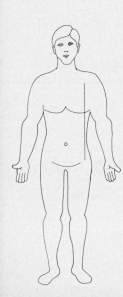

1 Spleen
2 Heart
3 Fundus of the stomach
4 Diaphragm
5 Transverse colon
6 Pancreas
7 Splenic artery and vein
8 Left kidney
9 Small bowel
10 Sigmoid colon
11 Iliacus muscle
12 Obturator externus muscle

13 Gluteus maximus muscle
14 Obturator internus muscle
15 Gluteus medius muscle
16 Quadratus lumborum muscle

Pelvic Viscera in the Male

Fig. 214 CONTACT SURFACES OF THE ABDOMINAL VISCERA AS SEEN FROM THE LEFT

The posterior pelvic cavity is occupied by the rectum, colon, and ileum (Fig. 214). The anterior parts are occupied by the bladder, ureter, vasa deferentia, seminal vesicles, prostate, and prostate urethra (Fig. 215).

BLADDER

The urinary bladder lies posterior to the pubic bones. The empty bladder is pyramidal and has an apex, a base, a neck, and superior and inferolateral surfaces.

The superolateral angles of the base are joined by the ureters, and the inferior angle gives rise to the urethra. The vasa deferentia separate the seminal vesicles at the posterior surface of the bladder.

URETER

The ureter crosses the pelvic inlet anterior to the bifurcation of the common iliac artery. At the ischial spine it turns forward and medially and enters the lateral upper angle of the bladder. Near its termination, the vas deferens crosses it.

VAS DEFERENS

The vas deferens arises from the deep inguinal ring and passes the inferior epigastric artery. It crosses the ureter near the ischial spine, then runs posterior to the bladder. The terminal end is dilated to form the ampulla of the vas deferens. The inferior end of the ampulla narrows and joins the duct of the seminal vesicle to form the ejaculatory duct.

PROSTATE

The prostate is a fibromuscular and glandular organ that surrounds the prostatic urethra. It lies between the neck of the bladder and the urogenital diaphragm. It is surrounded by a fibrous capsule, which in turn is surrounded by a fibrous sheath (part of the visceral layer of the pelvic fascia).

The arterial supply to the prostate is from the inferior vesical and middle rectal arteries. The veins drain into the internal iliac veins.

The visceral pelvic fascia covers and supports the pelvic viscera. It is continuous with the fascia covering the levator ani and coccygeus muscles, and with the parietal pelvic fascia on the pelvic walls.

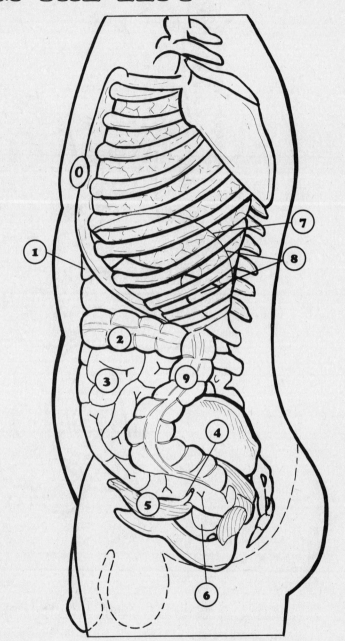

¹Liver
²Transverse colon
³Intestine
⁴Ureter
⁵Bladder
⁶Prostate
⁷Diaphragm
⁸Spleen
⁹Descending colon

Fig. 215 CORONAL SECTION OF THE MALE PELVIS

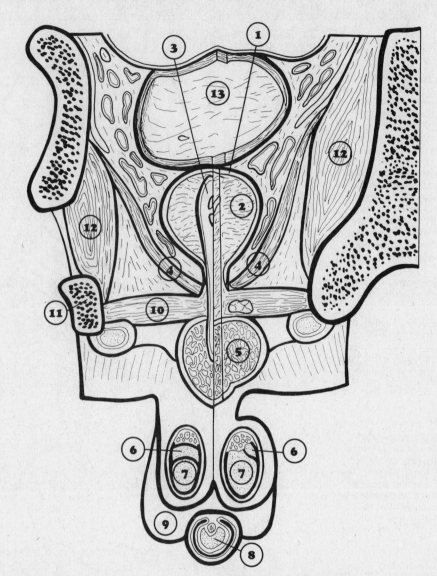

¹Ejaculatory duct
²Prostate
³Urethra
⁴Levator ani muscle
⁵Bulbous corpus cavernosum
⁶Epididymis
⁷Testis
⁸Corpus cavernosum penis

⁹Scrotum
¹⁰Tranverse perineal muscle
¹¹Pubis
¹²Obturator internus muscle
¹³Urinary bladder

Fig. 216 PERINEAL MUSCLES AND FLOOR OF THE PELVIS

MALE UROGENITAL TRIANGLE

Superficial Perineal Pouch

The superficial perineal pouch contains structures that form the root of the penis and their surrounding muscles. The root of the penis is made up of three masses of erectile tissue: the bulb of the penis and the right and left crura. The bulb is in the midline and is attached to the urogenital diaphragm. The urethra traverses it. The outer surface is covered by the bulbocavernous muscles. The crura are attached to the pubic arch and covered by the ischiocavernous muscles. The bulb projects forward into the body of the penis to form the corpus spongiosum. The two crura converge in the posterior body to form the corpora cavernosa. The superficial transverse perineal muscles lie in the posterior superficial perineal pouch. They serve to maintain the perineal body in the center of the perineum.

Several muscles are attached to the perineal body (Fig. 216):

The external and sphincter

The bulbospongiosus

The superficial transverse perineal

The perineal branch of the pudendal nerve terminates in the superficial perineal pouch.

Deep Perineal Pouch

The deep perineal pouch contains the membranous part of the urethra, the sphincter urethrae, the bulbourethral glands, the deep transverse perineal muscles, the internal pudendal vessels, and the dorsal nerves of the penis.

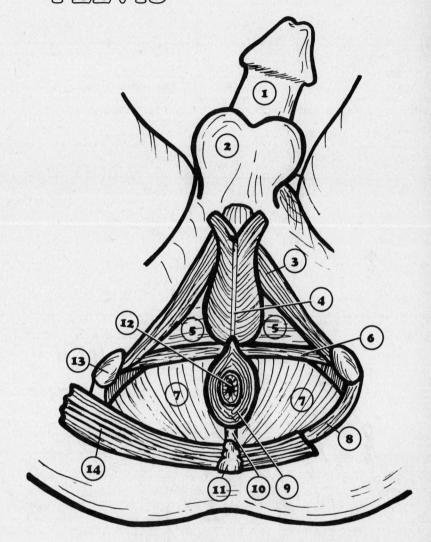

¹Penis
²Scrotum
³Ischiocavernosus muscle
⁴Bulbospongiosus muscle
⁵Urogenital diaphragm
⁶Transverse perineal muscle
⁷Levator ani muscle
⁸Sacrotuberous ligament
⁹Sphincter ani externus muscle
¹⁰Anococcygeal ligament
¹¹Coccyx
¹²Anus
¹³Ischial tuberosity
¹⁴Gluteus maximus muscle

Fig. 217 SAGITTAL VIEW OF THE MALE PELVIS

SCROTUM

The scrotum is really an outpouch of the lower abdominal wall. It contains the testes, the epididymides, and the lower ends of the spermatic cords (Fig. 217).

The superficial fascia is continuous with the fatty and membranous layers of the anterior abdominal wall. The fat is replaced by the smooth dartos muscle.

Both layers of superficial fascia contribute to a partition that crosses the scrotum and separates the testes from each other. The spermatic fascia lie underneath the superficial fascia and are derived from the layers of the anterior abdominal wall.

The tunica vaginalis covers the anterior, medial, and lateral surfaces of each testis. The testis is a mobile organ within the scrotum. The left testis is usually lower than the right. Each is surrounded by a tough fibrous capsule, the tunica albuginea.

The epididymis lies posterior to the testis, with the vas deferens on its medial side. The testis is connected to the head of the epididymis by the efferent ductules.

URETHRA

The male urethra extends from the neck of the bladder to the external meatus on the glans penis. It has three parts: prostatic, membranous, and penile.

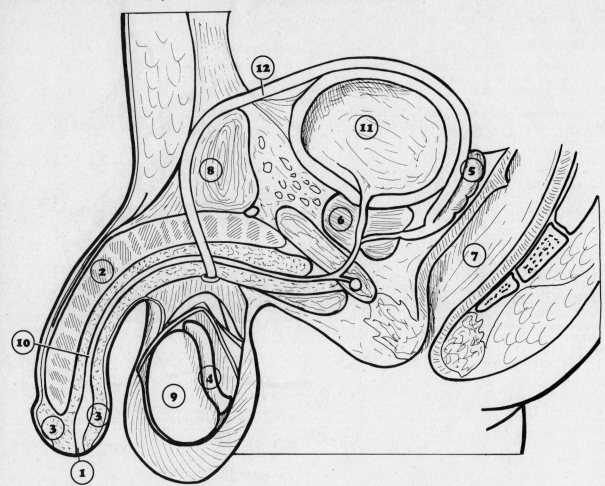

¹Bulb of the urethra
²Corpus cavernosum penis
³Corpus spongiosum penis
⁴Epididymis
⁵Seminal vesicle
⁶Prostate gland
⁷Rectum
⁸Symphysis pubis
⁹Testis
¹⁰Urethra
¹¹Urinary bladder
¹²Ductus deferens

Fig. 218 PELVIC CROSS SECTION, LEVEL 1

SERIAL CROSS SECTIONS OF THE MALE PELVIS

Level 1 (Fig. 218)

This section is taken at the level of the fifth lumbar vertebra. It cuts the ilium through the upper part of the iliac fossa and passes just above the wings of the sacrum. The gluteus medius and iliacus muscles are shown. The right common iliac artery bifurcates into the external and internal iliac arteries. The common iliac veins are shown to unite to form the inferior vena cava. The lower part of the greater omentum is shown in this section.

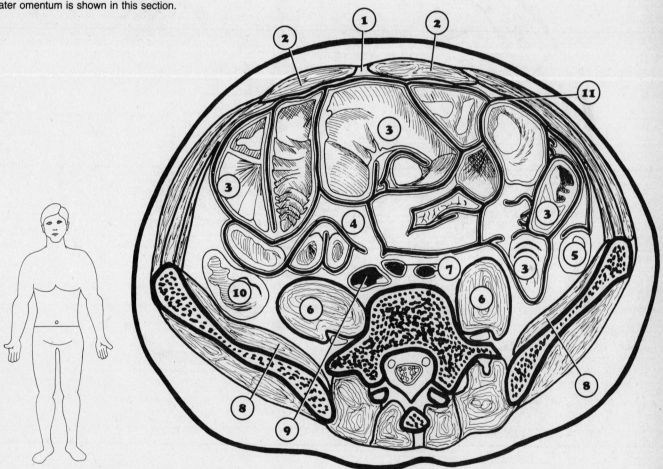

¹Linea alba	⁶Psoas major muscle
²Rectus abdominis muscle	⁷Iliac artery
	⁸Iliacus muscle
³Ileum	⁹Inferior vena cava
⁴Mesentery	¹⁰Ascending colon
⁵Descending colon	¹¹Peritoneal cavity

Fig. 219 PELVIC CROSS SECTION, LEVEL 2

Level 2 (Fig. 219)

Level 2 (Fig. 219)

This section is taken at the lower margin of the fifth lumbar vertebra and disc. The gluteus minimus muscle is shown on this section as are the right external and internal iliac arteries. The left common iliac artery branches into the external and internal arteries. The ileum is seen throughout this level, and the mesentery terminates at this level.

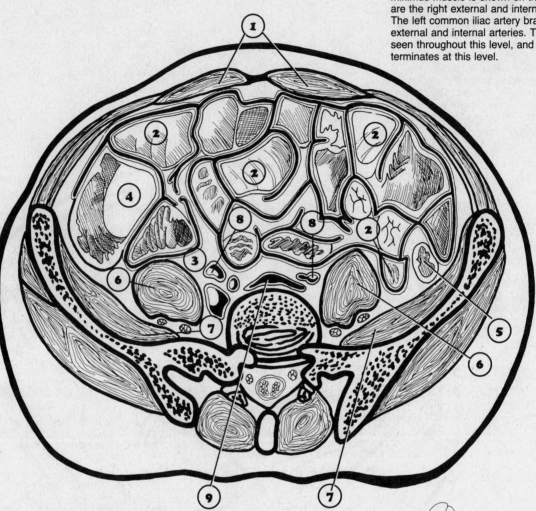

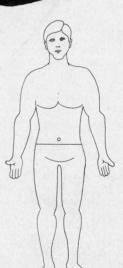

¹Rectus abdominis muscle
²Ileum
³Mesentery
⁴Ascending colon
⁵Descending colon
⁶Psoas major muscle
⁷Iliacus muscle
⁸External iliac artery
⁹Iliac vein

Fig. 220 PELVIC CROSS SECTION, LEVEL 3

Level 3 (Fig. 220)

This section is taken at the level of the sacrum and the anterior superior spine of the ilium. The gluteus maximus muscle appears on both sides. The internal and external iliac veins have united to form the common iliac vein. The ileum is seen throughout this section.

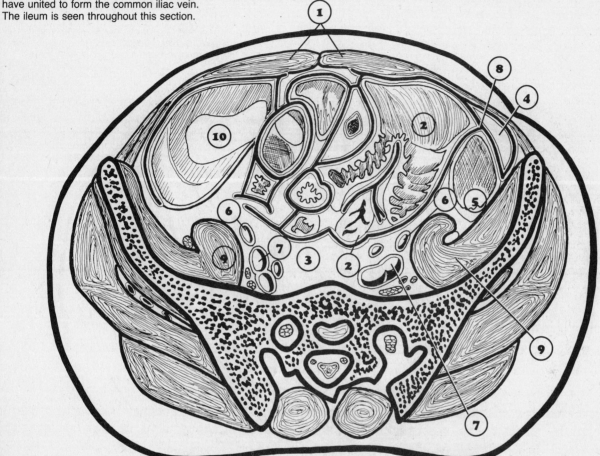

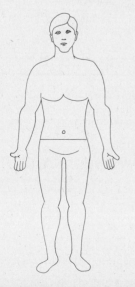

[1] Rectus abdominis muscle
[2] Ileum
[3] Mesentery
[4] Greater omentum
[5] Descending colon
[6] External iliac artery
[7] External iliac vein
[8] Peritoneal cavity
[9] Iliopsoas muscle
[10] Ascending colon

Fig. 221 PELVIC CROSS SECTION, LEVEL 4

Level 4 (Fig. 221)

This section passes through the third sacral vertebra near the upper margin of the third anterior sacral foramina. The pyramidalis, obturatorius internus, and piriformis muscles are shown. The cecum is also seen in this section. The lower portion of the descending colon passes over the sigmoid colon, and the sigmoid colon passes over into the rectum.

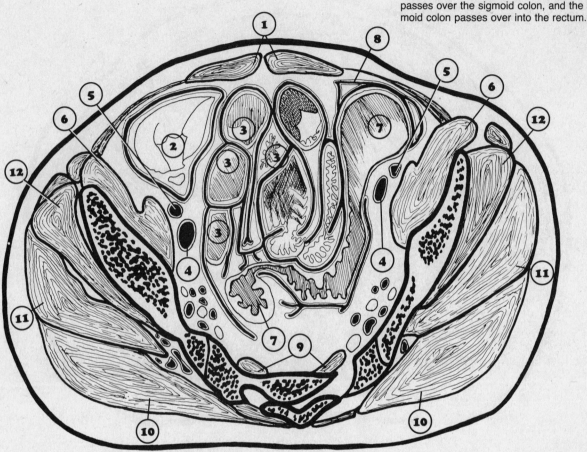

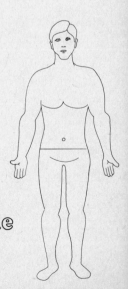

¹Rectus abdominis muscle

²Cecum

³Ileum

⁴External iliac vein

⁵External iliac artery

⁶Iliopsoas muscle

⁷Sigmoid colon

⁸Peritoneal cavity

⁹Piriformis muscle

¹⁰Gluteus maximus muscle

¹¹Gluteus medius muscle

¹²Gluteus minimus muscle

Fig. 222 PELVIC CROSS SECTION, LEVEL 5

Level 5 (Fig. 222)

This section passes through the sacrum above the margins of the fifth anterior pair of sacral foramina, through the acetabulum and the head of the femur. The external iliac arteries become the femoral arteries in this section. The femoral veins become the external iliac veins. The cecum and rectum are seen. The upper surface of the bladder, the ureters, the seminal vesicles, and the spermatic cord are well visualized.

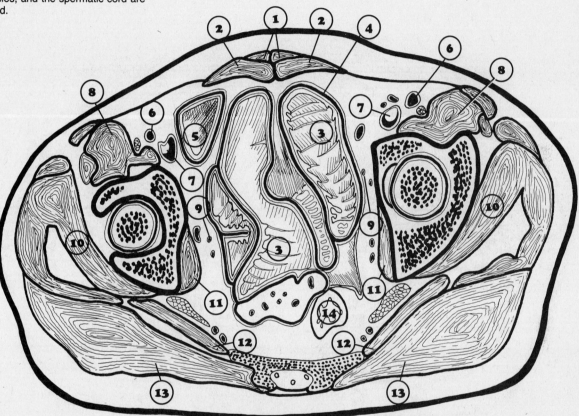

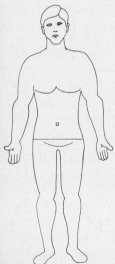

¹**Pyramidalis muscle**
²**Rectus abdominis muscle**
³**Ileum**
⁴**Peritoneal cavity**
⁵**Cecum**
⁶**External iliac artery**
⁷**External iliac vein**
⁸**Iliopsoas muscle**
⁹**Ductus deferens**
¹⁰**Gluteus minimus muscle**
¹¹**Obturator internus muscle**
¹²**Piriformis muscle**
¹³**Gluteus maximus muscle**
¹⁴**Rectum**

Fig. 223 PELVIC CROSS SECTION, LEVEL 6

Level 6 (Fig. 223)

This section passes through the coccyx, the spine of the ischium, the acetabulum, the head of the femur, the greater trochanter, the pubic symphysis, and the upper margins of the obturator foramen. The gemellus inferior and superior, coccygeus, and levator ani muscles are shown. The rectum is seen in the midline. The trigone of the bladder and the urethral orifice are well shown, and the seminal vesicles and the ampulla of the vasa deferentia can be identified. The ejaculatory ducts enter the urethra in the lower portion of this section. Also shown is the prostate gland.

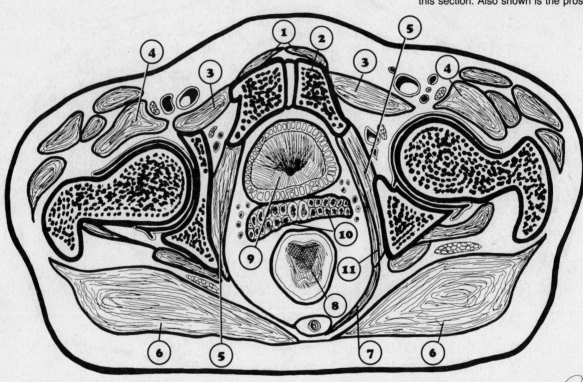

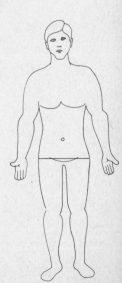

1 Pyramidalis muscle
2 Pubic os
3 Pectineus muscle
4 Iliopsoas muscle
5 Obturator internus muscle
6 Gluteus maximus muscle
7 Coccygeus muscle
8 Rectum
9 Bladder
10 Seminal vesicles
11 Levator ani muscle

Fig. 224 PELVIC CROSS SECTION, LEVEL 7

Level 7 (Fig. 224)

This section passes below the tip of the coccyx, the upper portion of the tuberosity of the ischium and of the inferior ramus of the pubis, the neck of the femur, and the lower portion of the greater trochanter. The ischiocavernosus, adductor brevis and longus, and the obturator internus muscles are seen. The rectum, prostate gland, penis, and corpus cavernosum are also seen on this section.

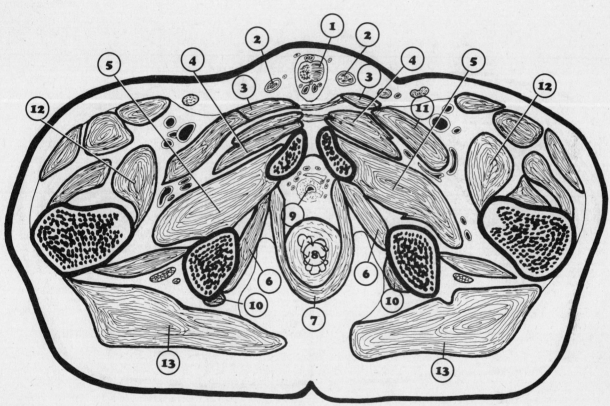

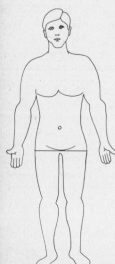

1 Penile fascia
2 Ductus deferens
3 Adductor longus muscle
4 Adductor brevis muscle
5 Obturator externus muscle
6 Obturator internus muscle
7 Levator ani muscle
8 Anus
9 Rectum
10 Ischiocavernous muscle
11 Pectineus muscle
12 Iliopsoas muscle
13 Gluteus maximus muscle

237

Fig. 225 PELVIC CROSS SECTION, LEVEL 8

Level 8 (Fig. 225)

This section passes through the inferior ramus of the pubis, the ramus of the ischium, and the femur at the level of the middle of the lesser trochanter. Thses muscles are seen: the sphincter ani internus, the bulbocavernosus, and the cremaster. The following muscles end in this section: quadratus femoris, sphincter ani externus and internus, levator ani, ischiocavernosus, obturator externus, and iliopsoas. The section passes through the root and body of the penis.

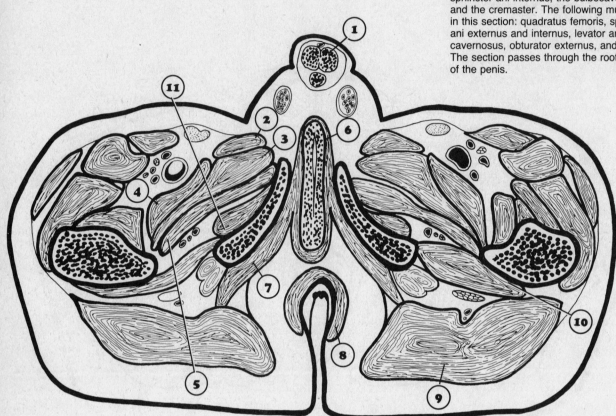

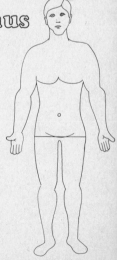

¹Corpus cavernosum penis

²Adductor longus muscle

³Adductor brevis muscle

⁴Pectineus muscle

⁵Adductor minimus muscle

⁶Crus penis

⁷Ischiocavernous muscle

⁸Sphincter ani internus muscle

⁹Gluteus maximus muscle

¹⁰Quadratus femoris muscle

¹¹Obturator externus muscle

Fig. 226 PELVIC CROSS SECTION, LEVEL 9

Level 9 (Fig. 226)

This section passes through the femur, the scrotum, the upper portion of the left testicle, and the epididymis. The lining membrane and tunica vaginalis of the scrotal cavity are seen as are the vas deferens and the vascular plexus.

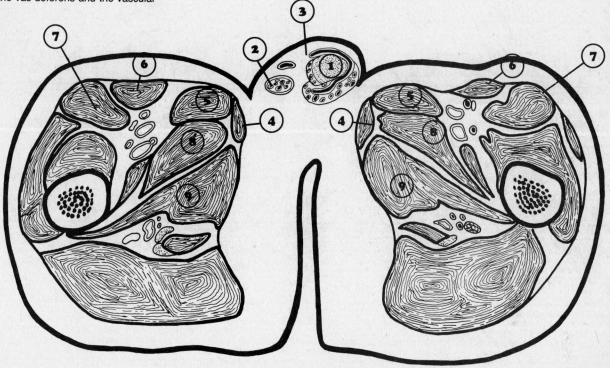

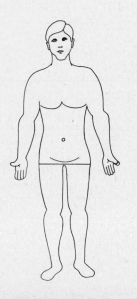

¹Testis
²Plexus pampiniformis
³Scrotum
⁴Gracilis muscle
⁵Adductor longus muscle
⁶Sartorius muscle
⁷Rectus femoris muscle
⁸Adductor brevis muscle
⁹Adductor minimus muscle

Fig. 227 SAGITTAL SECTION OF THE MALE PELVIS, LEVEL 1

SERIAL SAGITTAL
SECTIONS OF THE MALE
PELVIS (Figs. 227 Through
229)

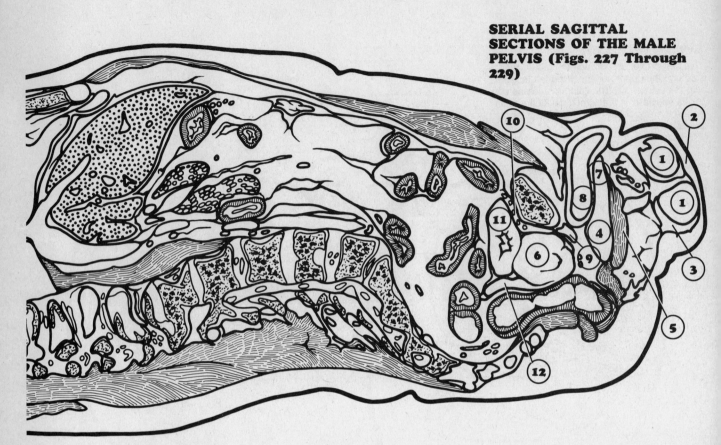

1 Testis
2 Scrotum
3 Epididymis
4 Bulb of the penis
5 Bulbospongiosus
   muscle
6 Prostate
7 Corpus spongiosum
   penis
8 Corpus cavernosum
   penis
9 Crus of the penis
10 Retropubic space
11 Bladder
12 Seminal vesicles

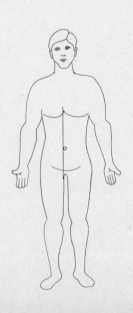

Fig. 228 SAGITTAL SECTION OF THE MALE PELVIS, LEVEL 2

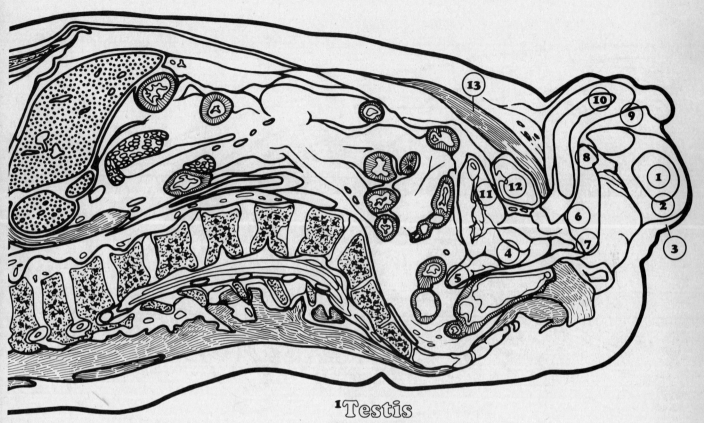

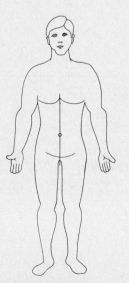

1 Testis
2 Epididymis
3 Scrotum
4 Prostate
5 Seminal vesicles
6 Bulb of the penis
7 Bulbospongiosus muscle
8 Corpus spongiosum penis
9 Glans penis
10 Corpus cavernosum penis
11 Bladder
12 Symphysis pubis
13 Pyramidalis muscle

Fig. 229 SAGITTAL SECTION OF THE MALE PELVIS, LEVEL 3

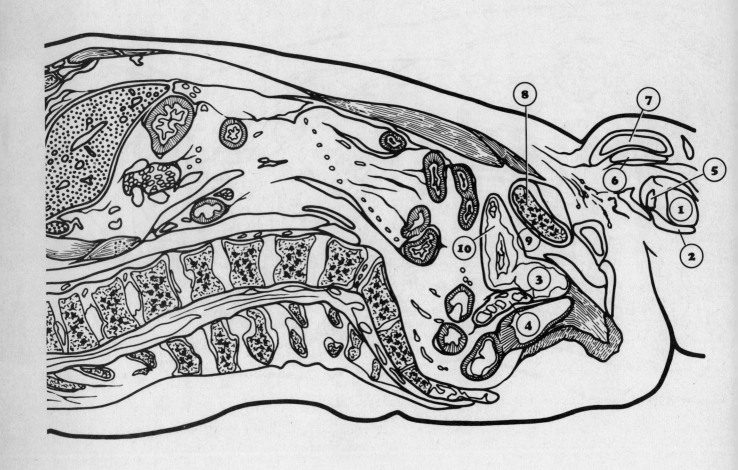

¹Testis
²Head of the epididymis
³Prostate
⁴Seminal vesicle
⁵Plexus pampiniformis
⁶Corpus spongiosum
   penis
⁷Corpus cavernosum
   penis
⁸Body of the pubis
⁹Retropubic space
¹⁰Bladder

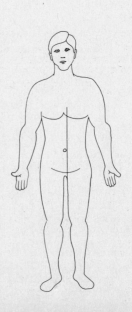

Pelvic Viscera in the Female

Fig. 230 THORACIC LANDMARKS AND ABDOMINAL-PELVIC VISCERA AS SEEN FROM THE RIGHT

The posterior part of the pelvic cavity is occupied by the rectum, colon, and ileum. The anterior pelvic cavity contains the bladder, ureters, ovaries, fallopian tubes, uterus, and vagina (Fig. 230).

BLADDER

The apex of the bladder is located posterior to the pubic bones, its base is anterior to the vagina, and the superior surface is related to the uterus. Its neck rests on the upper surface of the urogenital diaphragm. The inferolateral surfaces relate to the retropubic fat, the pubic bones, and the obturator internus and levator ani muscles.

URETER

The ureter crosses the pelvic inlet anterior to the bifurcation of the common iliac artery. It runs in front of the internal iliac artery and posterior to the ovary to the ischial spine. It turns forward and medially, under the base of the broad ligament where it is crossed by the uterine artery. The ureter runs forward, lateral to the vagina, to enter the bladder.

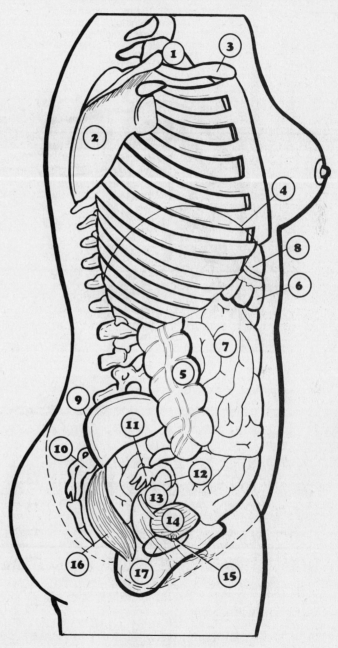

1 Apex of the lung
2 Scapula
3 Clavicle
4 Diaphragm
5 Ascending colon
6 Transverse colon
7 Intestine
8 Stomach
9 Posterior iliac spine
10 Sacral os
11 Infundibulum (uterine tube)
12 Ovary
13 Uterus
14 Bladder
15 Urethra
16 Rectum
17 Vagina

Fig. 231 OVARY AND BROAD LIGAMENT

OVARY

Each small, almond-shaped ovary is attached to the back of the broad ligament by the mesovarium, sometimes called the suspensory ligament of the ovary (Fig. 231).

The round ligament of the ovary extends from the upper end of the lateral wall of the uterus to the medial margin of the ovary. The ovary lies in the ovarian fossa. The fossa is bounded by the external iliac vessels, ureter, and obturator nerve. The position of the ovary varies.

The ovary receives its blood supply from the ovarian artery. The ovarian vein drains into the inferior vena cava on the right and into the left renal vein on the left.

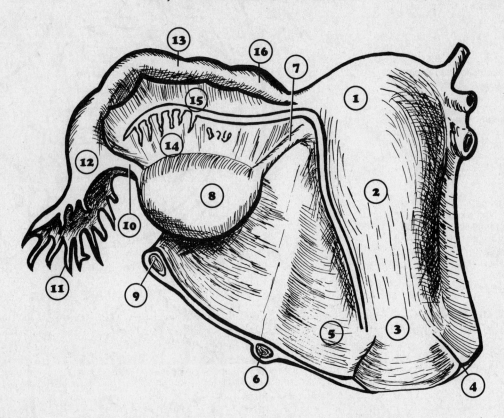

¹Fundus of the uterus
²Body of the uterus
³Cervix of the uterus
⁴Uterosacral fold and ligament
⁵Broad ligament
⁶Ligamentum teres
⁷Ovarian ligament
⁸Ovary
⁹Suspensory ligament of the ovary
¹⁰Fimbria ovarica
¹¹Fimbriae
¹²Infundibulum
¹³Ampulla of the fallopian tube
¹⁴Mesovarium
¹⁵Mesosalpinx
¹⁶Isthmus of the fallopian tube

Fig. 232 FEMALE PELVIS AS VIEWED FROM ABOVE

FALLOPIAN TUBES

The long, slender fallopian tubes lie along the upper border of the broad ligament. They connect the peritoneal cavity to the uterine cavity. The tube is divided into four parts: the infundibulum, the ampulla, the isthmus, and the interstice (Fig. 232).

The infundibulum is the funnel-shaped lateral extremity that projects beyond the broad ligament to overlie the ovaries. The free edge of the funnel has a number of fingerlike processes (fimbriae) draped over the ovary.

The ampulla is the widest part of the tube. The isthmus is the narrowest part and lies just lateral to the uterus. The interstice of the tube pierces the uterine wall.

The ovarian arteries and veins are the vascular supply to the tube.

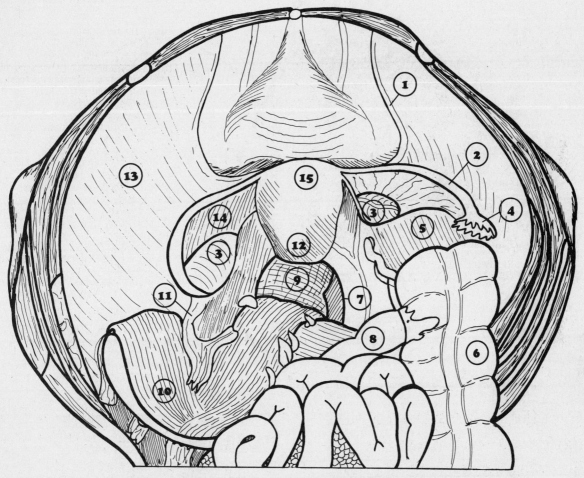

¹Ligamentum teres uteri	⁹Pouch of Douglas
²Fallopian tube	¹⁰Sigmoid colon
³Ovary	¹¹Ovarian suspensory ligament
⁴Fimbriae	
⁵Ovarian fossa	¹²Cervix
⁶Ascending colon	¹³Iliac fossa
⁷Rectouterine surface	¹⁴Mesosalpinx
⁸Ileum	¹⁵Vesicouterine surface

Fig. 233 SAGITTAL SECTION OF THE FEMALE PELVIS

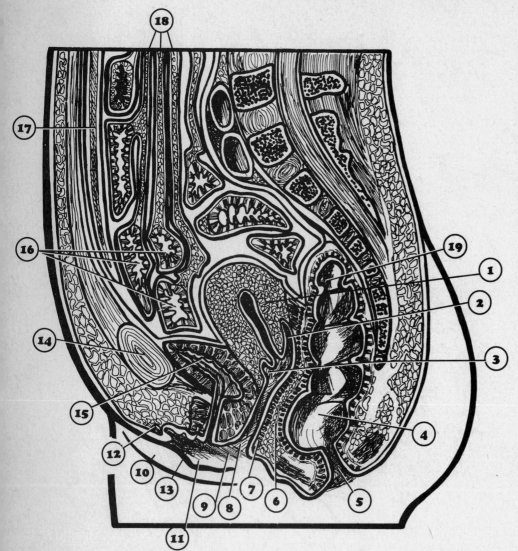

UTERUS

The uterus is a hollow, pear-shaped organ with very thick muscular walls. It is divided into the fundus, body, and cervix.

The cavity of the uterine body is funnel shaped on a coronal plane but merely a slit on a sagittal plane (Fig. 233). The cavity of the cervix, the cervical canal, communicates with the uterine cavity by the internal os and to the vagina by the external os.

The uterus is generally anteflexed and anteverted in the pelvis. It is covered with peritoneum except anteriorly, below the internal os, where peritoneum is reflected onto the bladder. There is also a lateral space between the layers of the broad ligament.

The muscular wall, or myometrium, is a thick, smooth muscle supported by connective tissue. The endometrium is the mucous membrane of the uterine body.

The body of the uterus is related anteriorly to the uterovesical pouch and the superior surface of the bladder. Posteriorly it relates to the rectouterine pouch (the pouch of Douglas), the ileum, and the colon. Laterally the body of the uterus is related to the broad ligament and uterine vessels.

The arterial supply is from the uterine artery, a branch of the internal iliac artery. The uterine vein drains into the internal iliac vein.

The uterus is supported by the levator ani muscles and the pelvic fascia, which form three important ligaments: the transverse cervical, the pubocervical, and the sacrocervical. The round ligament helps to keep the uterus anteflexed and anteverted.

¹Uterus
²Posterior fornix
³Anterior fornix
⁴Rectum
⁵Anal canal
⁶Rectovaginal septum
⁷Perineal body
⁸Vagina
⁹Vestibule of the vagina
¹⁰Labium majus

¹¹Labium minus
¹²Clitoris
¹³Urethra
¹⁴Pubic symphysis
¹⁵Urinary bladder
¹⁶Coils of the ileum
¹⁷Greater omentum
¹⁸Folds of the mesentery
¹⁹Sigmoid colon

Fig. 234 FEMALE PELVIS AS VIEWED FROM BELOW

VAGINA

The vagina extends upward and backward from the vulva. The upper half of the vagina lies above the pelvic floor, the lower half with the perineum. The area of the vaginal lumen surrounding the cervix is divided into four fornices (Fig. 234).

The arterial supply is from the vaginal and uterine arteries. The vaginal drains into the internal iliac vein.

PELVIC VISCERAL FASCIA

The pelvic visceral fascia is a layer of connective tissue that covers and supports the pelvic viscera. It forms the pubocervical, transverse cervical, and sacrocervical ligaments of the uterus. The fascia in the uterine region is referred to as the parametrium. The visceral fascia is continuous with the fascia covering the levator ani and coccygeus muscles, and on the pelvic walls with the parietal pelvic fascia.

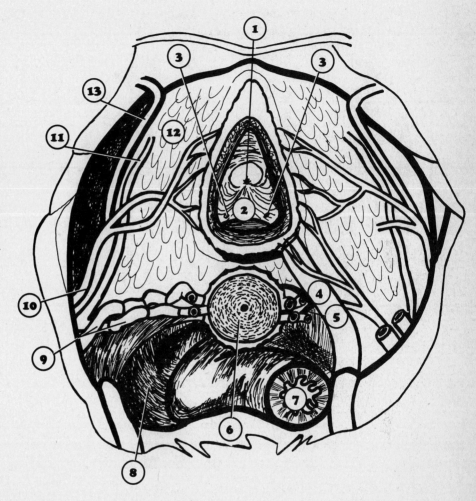

¹Urethral opening
²Trigone of the bladder
³Openings of the ureters
⁴Ureter
⁵Vaginal artery
⁶Cervix
⁷Rectum

⁸Uterosacral ligament
⁹Uterine vein and artery
¹⁰Superior vesical artery
¹¹Obturator artery
¹²Subserous fascia
¹³Obliterated umbilical artery

Fig. 235 MUSCLES OF THE FEMALE PELVIS

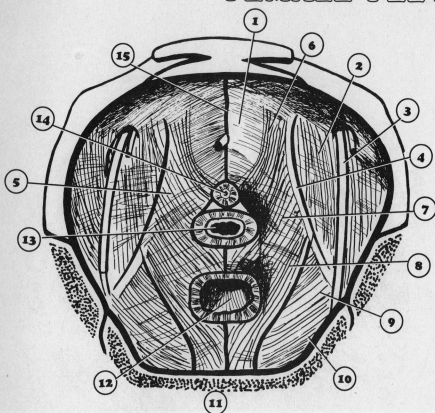

¹Pubic bone
²Obturator internus muscle
³Obturator nerve and artery
⁴Arcus tendineus
⁵Levator ani muscle:
    ⁶Pubovaginalis muscle
    ⁷Puborectalis muscle
    ⁸Pubococcygeus muscle
    ⁹Iliococcygeus muscle
¹⁰Coccygeus muscle
¹¹Sacrum
¹²Rectum
¹³Vagina
¹⁴Urethra
¹⁵Deep fascia (cut edge)

FEMALE UROGENITAL TRIANGLE

Superficial Perineal Pouch

The superficial perineal pouch contains the structures that form the root of the clitoris and its surrounding muscles. The root of the clitoris is composed of three masses of erectile tissue: the bulb of the vestibule and the right and left crura of the clitoris. The bulb of the vestibule is divided into halves. It is attached to the urogenital diaphragm and is covered by bulbospongiosus muscles. The halves unite anteriorly to form the glans clitoris.

The crura of the clitoris are covered by the ischiocavernous muscles. The superficial transverse perineal muscles are the same as in the male.

The perineal body is a wedge-shaped mass of fibrous tissue that lies between the vagina and the anal canal. Many muscles, including the levator ani (which supports the posterior wall of the vagina), attach to its surface (Fig. 235).

The perineal branch of the pudendal nerve terminates in the superficial perineal pouch.

Deep Perineal Pouch

The deep perineal pouch contains part of the urethra, part of the vagina, the sphincter urethrae, the deep transverse perineal muscles, the internal pudendal vessels, and the dorsal nerves of the clitoris.

Vulva

The vulva is the female external genitalia. The mons pubis is composed of an underlying pad of fat.

The labia majora (equivalent to the scrotum) are prominent hair-bearing folds of skin extending from the mons pubis to unite posteriorly in the midline.

The labia minora are smaller folds of skin that lie between the labia majora. Their posterior ends unite to form a sharp fold, the fourchette. Anteriorly they split to enclose the clitoris.

The vestibule is a smooth, triangular area bounded by the labia minora, the clitoris, and the fourchette. The urethra and vagina perforate its surface.

The vaginal orifice is protected by the thin mucosal fold of the hymen.

The greater vestibular glands lie under the bulb of the vestibule and the labia majora.

The clitoris (corresponding to the penis in the male) is located at the apex of the vestibule.

Fig. 236 PELVIC CROSS SECTION, LEVEL 6

SERIAL CROSS SECTIONS OF THE FEMALE PELVIS

Level 6 (Fig. 236)

The section is taken just below the junction of the sacrum and coccyx, through the anterior inferior spine of the ilium and the great sciatic notch. The uterine artery and vein and the ureter are shown dissected beyond the uterine wall. The bladder is shown just anterior to the uterus, and the round ligament is shown. The ovaries are cut through their midsections on this level.

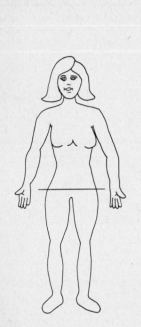

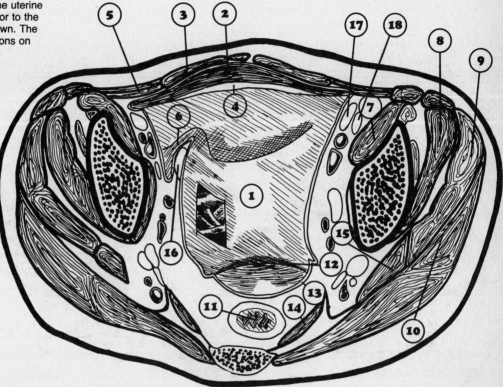

¹Uterus
²Pyramidalis muscle
³Rectus abdominis muscle
⁴Peritoneal cavity
⁵Obturator internus muscle
⁶Fallopian tube
⁷Iliopsoas muscle
⁸Gluteus minimus muscle

⁹Gluteus medius muscle
¹⁰Gluteus maximus muscle
¹¹Rectum
¹²Pouch of Douglas
¹³Peritoneum
¹⁴Coccygeus muscle
¹⁵Piriformis muscle
¹⁶Ovary
¹⁷External iliac vein
¹⁸External iliac artery

Fig. 237 PELVIC CROSS SECTION, LEVEL 7

Level 7 (Fig. 237)

This section is taken through the lower part of the coccyx and the spine of the ischium, the middle of the acetabulum, and the head of the femur. The superior gemellus muscles and the pectineus muscle appear in this section, and the coccygeus muscle terminates here. The gluteus maximus, gluteus minimus, and gluteus medius muscles all begin their insertions in the lower part of this section. The external os of the cervix is shown. The ureters empty into the bladder at the base.

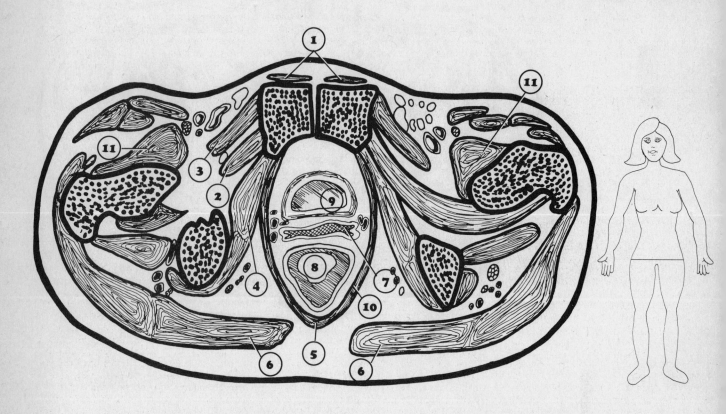

[1] Pyramidalis muscle
[2] Obturator externus muscle
[3] Pectineus muscle
[4] Obturator internus muscle
[5] Fascia of the pelvic diaphragm

[6] Gluteus maximus muscle
[7] Vagina
[8] Rectum
[9] Bladder
[10] Levator ani muscle
[11] Iliopsoas muscle

Female Reproductive Cycle

Fig. 238 EARLY CHANGES IN THE INTERRELATIONSHIPS OF EMBRYO AND EXTRAEMBRYONIC MEMBRANES: 4-WEEK GESTATION

IMPLANTATION AND FERTILIZATION

Approximately 14 days prior to a woman's next expected menstrual period, a matured ovarian follicle ruptures and releases an ovum into the peritoneal cavity. Very shortly after its release, the ovum is swept by the waving, fan-like motion of the fingerlike processes (fimbriae) of the fallopian tube into the lumen of the tube, where fertilization will later occur.

Once the ovum is within the fallopian tube, it is slowly moved along toward the uterus by the movement of the cillia that line the uterine tube as well as by smooth muscle contraction in the wall of the tube.

Fertilization must occur within 24 hours, since the ovum begins to degenerate after that time. The process of fertilization usually occurs within the ampulla of the uterine tube.

It usually takes approximately 3 days for the ovum to traverse the entire uterine tube, and the ovum has already begun its development by the time that it reaches the uterine cavity.

Unlike the ovum, the spermatozoa are self-propelled. Their moving tail acts in a fashion similar to that of the flagellum in the ovum. During coitus, several hundred million sperm are deposited in the vagina, and a great number of these quickly move through the cervical os and into the uterine tubes.

The movement of the sperm is probably assisted a great deal by the rhythmic contractions of the vagina, uterus, and uterine tubes. It has also been postulated that the prostaglandins found in the seminal fluid may aid in the stimulation of uterine contractions to aid in the upward travel of the sperm.

The fertilized ovum is termed a *zygote*. As the zygote travels, it also begins to divide to form a multicelled zygote. When the zygote reaches the uterine cavity, it prepares for implantation in the endometrial layer of the uterus. This usually occurs approximately 7 days after fertilization.

The site on the ovary from which the ovum came during ovulation becomes a site of active hormone secretion soon after fertilization. This ovarian follicle becomes the corpus luteum of pregnancy and produces progesterone, which is necessary for implantation of the zygote in the endometrium. The corpus luteum becomes unnecessary as the placenta develops to secrete sufficient quantities of progesterone.

The placenta serves as the major hormonal organ of pregnancy and secretes (among other things) chorionic gonadotrophin, which is necessary for the maintenance of the corpus luteum and is the hormone most often measured clinically as a test for pregnancy.

The placenta also produces the progesterone necessary for the maintenance of the uterine lining and the prevention of menstruation during pregnancy. The level of progesterone gradually increases during pregancy until the middle of the third trimester.

Various estrogens are also produced by the placenta. One of these estrogens, estriol, is produced by the placenta from precursors originating in the fetus. The measurement of the amount of estriol in maternal urine gives some index of uteroplacental function, and any precipitous drop in these levels may indicate a serious problem with the fetus or placenta.

THE PLACENTA

Soon after fertilization and implantation, the maternal endometrium, in response to the increased levels of progesterone and other hormones of pregnancy, undergoes a change in histology, forming a layer called the decidua. This layer has three parts: (1) the decidua basalis, which forms beneath the area of zygote implantation, (2) the decidua capsularis, which covers the implanted zygote, and (3) the decidua vera, which covers the remaining uterine cavity. The decidua basalis becomes the maternal contribution to the placenta and is sloughed off with it after delivery.

The zygote also differentiates into several parts. One part will become the embryo, while the other parts (extra-embryonic) will form the "fetal membranes" that form parts of the placenta. These membranes function in protection, nutrition, respiration and excretion of the embryo.

The yolk sac is the precursor of the alimentary canal (Fig. 238). The part of the yolk sac not used for gut formation gradually decreases in size and eventually becomes only a small vesicular remnant in the fetal side of the umbilical cord.

The amnion is formed from cells found on the interior of the developing cell mass that is to become the fetus and placenta (Fig. 239). The amnion becomes a thin, very tough transparent membrane enclosing the amniotic cavity. This cavity rapidly enlarges during development and impinges on the walls of the extra-embryonic cavity finally obliterating the cavity. The amnion fuses wtih the chorion and forms the set of membranes that enclose the amniotic fluid and fetus until delivery. The fetus produces the amniotic fluid contained within the cavity and constantly swallows and replaces it.

The amniotic fluid protects the fetus by providing a cusion or shock absorber, it provides room for movement, and it acts as a hydrostatic wedge during labor to dilate the cervix.

The chorion is derived from the outer layer of cells in the developing cell mass (Fig. 240). This layer is in direct contact with maternal tissue. The chorion fuses to the amnion layer to contribute to the amniotic cavity. It also becomes the complex network of vascular tissue that provides sufficient communication with maternal fluids to provide the fetus with nourishment and oxygen and to remove waste products.

¹Fetus
²Yolk sac
³Chorion
⁴Allantois
⁵Amnion
⁶Extraembryonic coelom

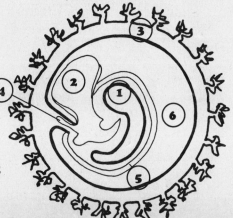

Fig. 239 6-WEEK GESTATION

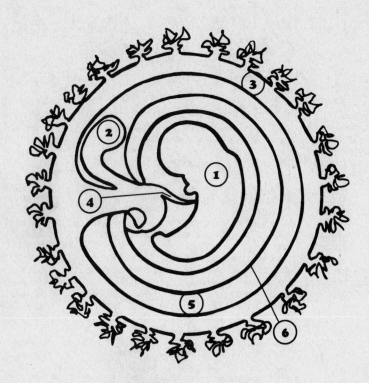

¹Fetus
²Yolk sac
³Chorion
⁴Allantois
⁵Extraembryonic coelom
⁶Amnion

Fig. 240 8-WEEK GESTATION

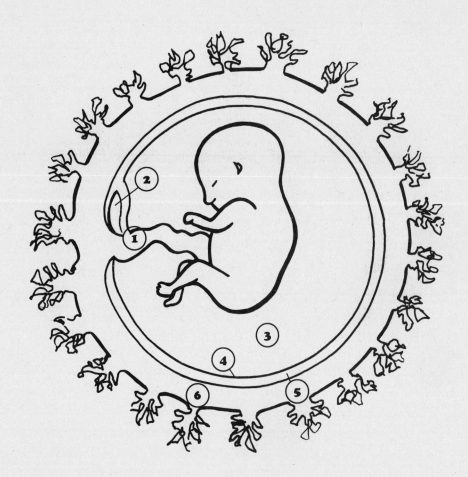

¹Umbilical cord
²Yolk sac
³Amniotic cavity
⁴Amnion
⁵Extraembryonic coelom
⁶Chorion

Female Breast

Fig. 241A CROSS SECTION OF THE FEMALE BREAST

The breast is a differentiated apocrine sweat gland. Its function is to secrete milk during lactation. Its parenchymal elements are the lobes, ducts, lobules, and acini (Fig. 241A). Because the mammary gland is a skin derivative, the stromal elements include dense connective tissue, loose connective tissue, and fat. The age and functional state of the breast dictate the amount and arrangement of the various parenchymal and stromal elements.

The breast is composed of 15 to 20 lobes. Each lobe contains the parenchymal elements of the breast. The ducts extend from the lobes through the breast parenchyma to converge in a single papilla (the nipple), which is surrounded by the areola. The ducts are covered with a connective tissue layer that varies in thickness and density. The normal duct usually measures approximately 2 mm in diameter.

The entire breast is enveloped in a duplication of superficial pectoral fascia (Fig. 241B). The posterior part of the fascia is connected to the pectoral musculature, the anterior part of the skin by thin connective tissue septa. The anterior and posterior fascial planes are connected by curvilinear connective tissue septa known as Cooper's ligaments. The connective tissue septa envelope the lobules and lobes of the breast and become the interlobular and interlobar connective tissues that surround the fat lobules and parenchyma of the breast.

There are three well-defined layers in the breast: subcutaneous, mammary, and retromammary. The subcutaneous layer is bounded superficially by the dermis and deeply by the superficial connective tissue plane. The principal component of the layer is fat lobules enclosed by connective tissue septa. The mammary layer is composed of breast parenchyma and is found between the superficial and deep connective tissue layers. Fat is seen to be interspersed in a lobular fashion throughout the entire breast parenchyma. The retromammary layer consists of fat lobules that are separated anteriorly from the mammary layer by the deep connective tissue plane and posteriorly by the fascia over the pectoralis major muscle.

During pregnancy the ducts and parenchymal elements of the breast expand to such a degree that the mammary layer constitutes almost the entire breast. The subcutaneous fat layer and the retromammary layer become squeezed together during this period.

The major portion of the breast contained within the superficial fascia of the anterior thoracic wall is situated between the second or third rib superiorly, the sixth or seventh costal cartilage inferiorly, and the sternal border medially. The greatest amount of glandular tissue is located in the upper outer quadrant of the breast, which explains why tumors are most frequently found here.

The major pectoral muscle lies posterior to the retromammary layer. The minor pectoral muscle lies superolaterally posterior to it. The pectoralis minor courses from its origin in the rib cage to the point where it inserts into the coracoid process. The lower border of the pectoralis major muscle forms the anterior border of the axilla. Breast tissue can extend into this region and is referred to as the axillary tail, or tail of Spence (Fig. 242).

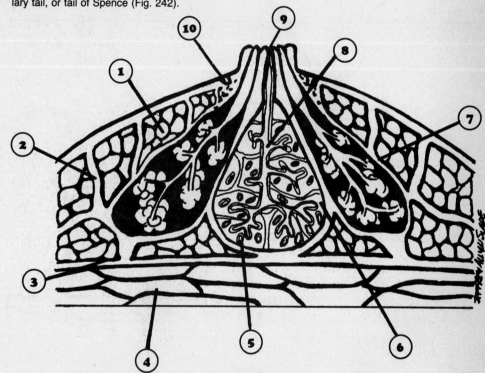

1 Subcutaneous fat
2 Cooper's ligaments
3 Retromammary layer
4 Pectoralis major muscle
5 Acinus
6 Interlobular connective tissue
7 Superficial fascia
8 Lactiferous duct
9 Ampulla
10 Montgomery's gland

Fig. 241B STRUCTURE OF THE FEMALE BREAST AS SEEN FROM ABOVE

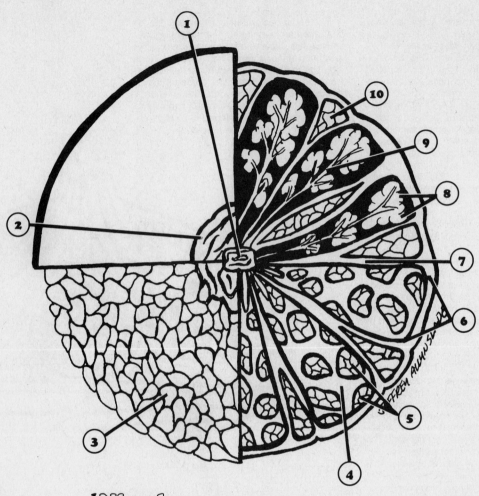

¹Nipple
²Areola
³Subcutaneous fat
⁴Interlobular connective
    tissue
⁵Lobules
⁶Lobe
⁷Cooper's ligaments
⁸Acini
⁹Lactiferous ducts
¹⁰Mammary fat

Fig. 242 AXILLARY TAIL (TAIL OF SPENCE)

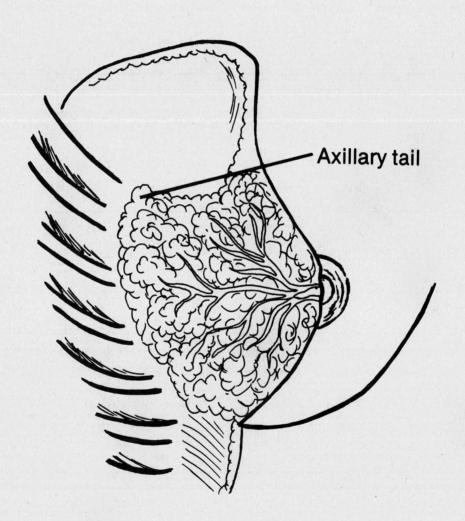

Axillary tail

Cranial Cavity

The brain and its surrounding meninges and portions of the cranial nerves, arteries, veins, and venous sinuses are found within the cranial cavity.

VAULT OF THE SKULL

The coronal, sagittal, and lambdoid sutures line the internal surface of the cranial vault. A middle sagittal groove houses the superior sagittal sinus. A small foramen transmits an emissary vein from the superior sagittal sinus and perforates the parietal bone at the side of the sagittal groove. The middle meningeal vessels pass through narrow grooves up the side of the skull to the vault.

BASE OF THE SKULL

The base of the skull is divided into three cranial fossae: anterior, middle, and posterior.

Anterior Cranial Fossa

The anterior cranial fossa houses the frontal lobe of the cerebral hemispheres. The frontal bone is the anterior boundary, and in the midline is a crest for the attachment of the falx cerebri. The lesser wing of the sphenoid is the posterior border. The medial end of the lesser wing of the sphenoid forms the anterior clinoid process, which gives attachment to the tentorium cerebelli. The median part of the anterior cranial fossa is limited posteriorly by the groove for the optic chiasm.

The floor of the fossa is formed by the ridged orbital plates of the frontal bone laterally and by the cribriform plate of the ethmoid medially. The crista galli is a projection of the ethmoid bone for the attachment of the falx cerebri.

Middle Cranial Fossa

The median part of the median cranial fossa is formed by the body of the sphenoid. The temporal lobes of the cerebral hemispheres are found on its lateral, concave borders.

Anteriorly the lesser wings of the sphenoid and posteriorly the superior borders of the petrous portion of the temporal bones bound the fossa. Laterally lie the squamous parts of the temporal bones, the greater wings of the sphenoid, and the parietal bones.

The floor of each lateral part of the fossa is formed by the greater wing of the sphenoid and the squamous and petrous parts of the temporal bone.

Posterior Cranial Fossa

The posterior fossa contains the parts of the hindbrain—the cerebellum, pons, and medulla oblongata.

MENINGES

The brain and spinal cord are surrounded by three meninges: the dura mater, the arachnoid mater, and the pia mater.

Dura Mater

The dura mater has two layers: the endosteal layer and the meningeal layer. The endosteal layer is periosteum that covers the interior surface of the skull.

The meningeal layer is a strong fibrous membrane covering the brain and continuing through the foramen magnum with the dura mater of the spinal cord.

The falx cerebri is a sickle-shaped fold of dura mater that lies in the midline between the two cerebral hemispheres. It is attached in front to the internal frontal crest and the crista galli. Posteriorly it blends in the midline with the upper surface of the tentorium cerebelli.

The tentorium cerebelli is a fold of dura mater that forms the roof over the posterior cranial fossa. It covers the upper surface of the cerebellum and supports the occipital lobes of the cerebral hemispheres. The tentorial notch is in front for the passage of the midbrain.

The falx cerebri and the falx cerebelli are attached to the upper and lower surfaces of the tentorium.

The falx cerebelli is a small, sickle-shaped fold of dura mater that is attached to the internal occipital crest and projects forward between the two cerebellar hemispheres.

The diaphragma sellae is a fold of dura mater that forms the roof for the sella turcica.

Many arteries supply the dura mater; however, one of the more important arteries is the middle meningeal artery.

Arachnoid Mater

The arachnoid mater is an impermeable membrane that covers the brain and lies between the pia mater internally and the dura mater externally. It is separated from the pia by the subarachnoid space (which is filled with cerebrospinal fluid).

The cerebrospinal fluid is produced by the choroid plexuses within the ventricular system of the brain. It moves from the ventricular system through three foramina in the roof of the fourth ventricle to enter the subarachnoid space.

Pia Mater

The pia mater is a vascular membrane that covers the gyri and descends into the deepest sulci. It also extends over the cranial nerves and fuses with their epineuria. The cerebral arteries carry a sheath of pia with them as they enter the brain substance.

Venous Blood Sinuses

The venous sinuses are situated between the layers of the dura mater. They have no endothelial layer, valves, or muscle tissue.

The superior sagittal sinus occupies the upper fixed border of the falx cerebri. The inferior sagittal sinus occupies the free lower margin of the falx cerebri. The straight sinus occupies the line of junction of the falx cerebri with the tentorium cerebelli. The paired transverse sinuses begin at the internal occipital protuberance. The sigmoid sinuses are a direct continuation of the transverse sinuses. The occipital sinus occupies the attached margin of the falx cerebelli. The cavernous sinuses are located in the middle cranial fossa on each side of the sphenoid bone. The anterior and posterior intercavernous sinuses run in the diaphragmatic sellae in front of and behind the stalk of the hypophysis cerebri. The superior and inferior petrosal sinuses are located on the borders of the petrous part of the temporal bone.

Hypophysis Cerebri

The hypophysis cerebri, or pituitary gland, is a very important endocrine gland. It is located in the hypophyseal fossa (the deepest part of the sella turcica of the sphenoid bone).

Fig. 243 STRUCTURE OF THE BRAIN

BRAIN

Cerebrum

The cerebrum is the largest part of the brain. It consists of two cerebral hemispheres connected by a mass of white matter called the corpus callosum (Fig. 243). The hemispheres extend from the frontal to the occipital bones above the anterior and middle cranial fossae, and posteriorly above the tentorium cerebelli. The hemispheres are separated by the longitudinal fissure, into which projects the falx cerebri.

The surface layer of the hemispheres is called the cortex and is composed of gray matter. The cerebral cortex is thrown into folds, or gyri, separated by fissures, or sulci. The sulci further divide the hemispheres into lobes: frontal, parietal, occipital, and temporal.

The lateral ventricle is located within the cerebral hemisphere. It communicates with the third ventricle through the interventricular foramen.

Diencephalon

The diencephalon consists of a dorsal thalamus and a ventral hypothalamus. The thalamus lies on either side of the third ventricle.

Midbrain

The midbrain is narrow and connects the forebrain to the hindbrain. It consists of two halves, called the cerebral peduncles. The narrow cavity of the midbrain is the cerebral aqueduct, which connects the third and fourth ventricles. The tectum is the part of the tegmentum behind the cerebral aqueduct; it has four small surface swellings, the superior and inferior colliculi.

The pineal body lies between the superior colliculi and is attached by a stalk to the region of the posterior wall of the third ventricle.

Hindbrain

The pons is found on the anterior surface of the cerebellum below the midbrain and above the medulla oblongata. The medulla oblongata connects the pons to the spinal cord. A median fissure is present on the anterior surface of the medulla, with the pyramids on each side.

The inferior cerebellar peduncles connect the medulla to the cerebellum.

The cerebellum lies in the posterior cranial fossa under the tentorium cerebelli. Its two hemispheres are connected by the vermis.

The cerebellum is connected to the midbrain by the superior cerebellar peduncles, to the pons by the middle cerebellar peduncles, and to the medulla by the inferior cerebellar peduncles.

The fourth ventricle is the cavity of the hindbrain. It is connected to the third ventricle by the cerebral aqueduct and below is continuous with the central canal of the spinal cord.

Ventricles

The ventricles include the two lateral ventricles, the third ventricle, and the fourth ventricle.

The largest cavities are the lateral ventricles, which are divided for anatomical study into four segments: frontal horn, body, occipital horn, and temporal horn. The frontal horn is divided posteriorly by the foramen of Monro from the body of the ventricle. The roof is formed by the corpus callosum, the septum pellucidum forms the medial wall, and the head of the caudate nucleus forms the lateral wall.

The body of the lateral ventricle extends from the foramen of Monro to the trigone, formed by the junction with the temporal and occipital horns posteriorly. The corpus callosum forms the roof, and the septum pellucidum forms the medial wall. The thalamus touches the inferior lateral ventricular wall, and the body of the caudate nucleus borders the superior wall.

The temporal horn extends anteriorly from the trigone through the temporal lobe. The roof is formed by the white matter of the temporal lobe and by the tail of the caudate nucleus. The hippocampus forms the medial wall.

The occipital horn extends posteriorly from the trigone. The occipital cortex and white matter form the medial wall. The corpus callosum forms the proximal roof and lateral wall.

The third ventricle is connected by the foramen of Monro to the lateral ventricles. The aqueduct of Sylvius connects the third and fourth ventricles. The medulla oblongata forms the floor of the ventricle, while the cerebellar vermis and the posterior medullary vellum form the roof.

SAGITTAL PLANE (ANTERIOR FONTANELLE)

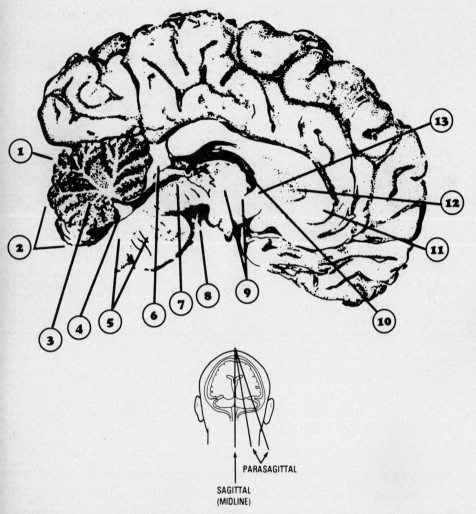

Sagittal (Midline)

1 Supracerebellar cistern
2 Cisterna magna
3 Vermis
4 Fourth ventricle
5 Brainstem
6 Quadrigeminal cistern
7 Aqueduct
8 Interpeduncular cistern
9 Third ventricle
10 Choroid plexus
11 Corpus callosum
12 Septum
13 Foramen of Monro

PARASAGITTAL

SAGITTAL
(MIDLINE)

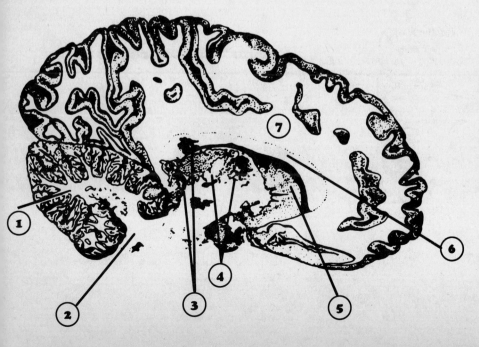

Parasagittal

1 Cerebellar hemisphere
2 Peduncle
3 Choroid plexus
4 Thalamus
5 Caudate nucleus
6 Lateral ventricle
7 Roof ventricle

CORONAL PLANE

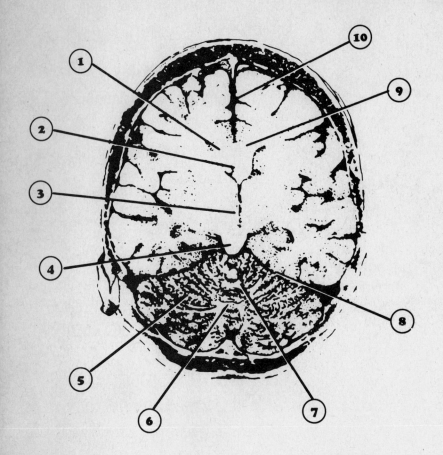

Modified Coronal (Anterior Fontanelle)

1. Lateral ventricle
2. Septum pellucidum
3. Third ventricle
4. Quadrigeminal cistern
5. Cerebellar hemisphere
6. Vermis
7. Fourth ventricle
8. Tentorium
9. Corpus callosum
10. Midline

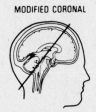

MODIFIED CORONAL

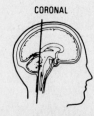

CORONAL

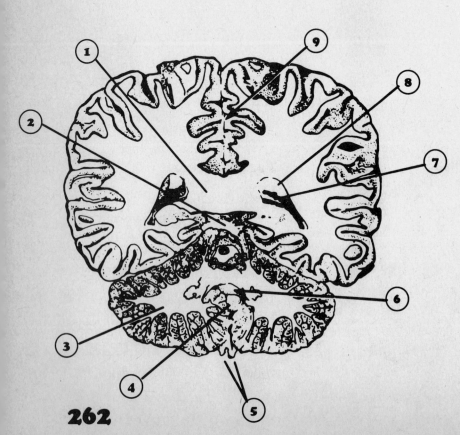

Coronal (Temporal Bone)

1. Corpus callosum
2. Quadrigeminal cistern
3. Cerebellar hemisphere
4. Vermis
5. Cisterna magna
6. Fourth ventricle
7. Choroid plexus
8. Lateral ventricle
9. Midline

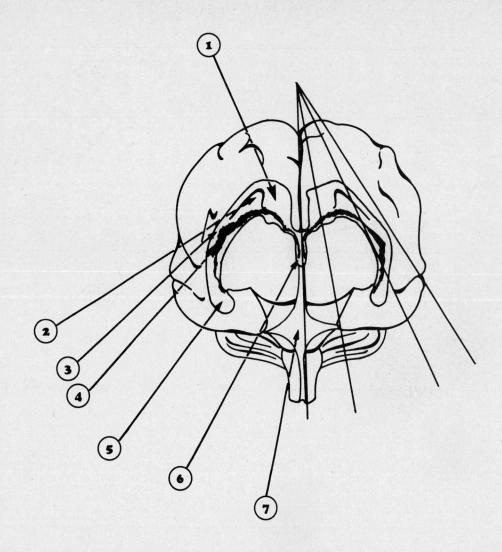

Coronal*

[1] Anterior horn
[2] Body of the lateral ventricle
[3] Atrium
[4] Choroid plexus
[5] Inferior horn
[6] Third ventricle
[7] Fourth ventricle

The pie-shaped lines represent a theoretical ultrasound transducer pathway through the neonatal skull.

Fig. 244 CORONAL PLANE THROUGH THE SKULL

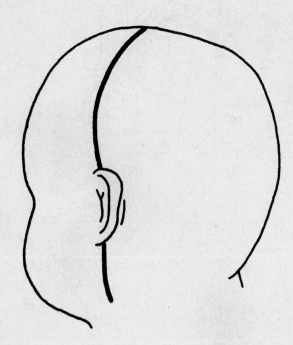

Sectional Anatomy

Coronal Section

The coronal section is obtained by looking at the brain 90° from the axial sections (Fig. 244). The anterior section of the brain shows the relationship of the frontal horns of the lateral ventricles to the caudate nuclei (Fig. 245). The caudate nuclei lie posterolateral to the frontal horn. The interhemispheric fissure is shown. As one moves slightly posterior, the cavum septi pellucidi is seen between the frontal horns (Fig. 246). Still more posterior are the thalami and the third ventricle (Fig. 247). The foramen of Monro may be seen in this section. The sylvian fissures are seen along each lateral wall of the brain. More posteriorly the pons and hippocampal gyrus are shown posterior to the bodies of the lateral ventricles and caudate nuclei (Fig. 248). The trigonum of the lateral ventricle and the choroid plexus is shown as it lies anterior to the cerebellum and tentorium (Fig. 249).

Fig. 245 CORONAL SECTION OF THE BRAIN THROUGH THE FRONTAL HORNS

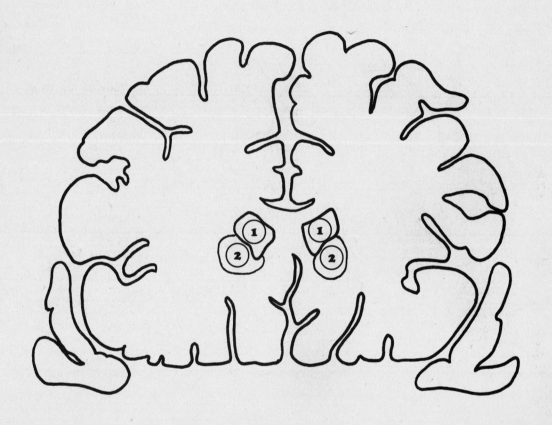

¹Frontal horn
²Caudate nucleus

Fig. 246 CORONAL SECTION OF THE BRAIN

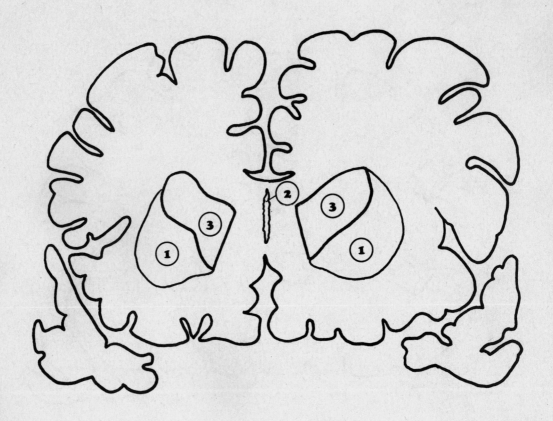

¹Caudate nucleus
²Cavum septi pellucidi
³Frontal horn

Fig. 247 CORONAL SECTION OF
THE BRAIN

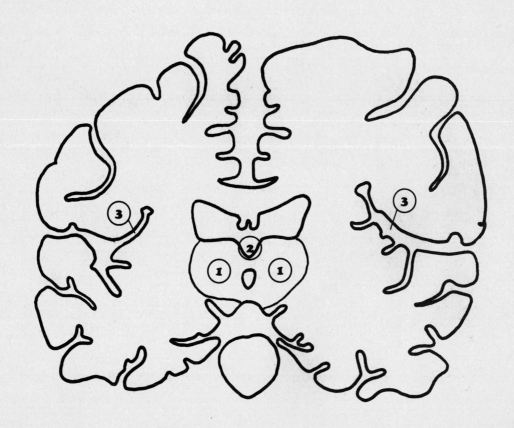

¹Thalamus
²Third ventricle
³Sylvian fissure

Fig. 248 CORONAL SECTION OF THE BRAIN

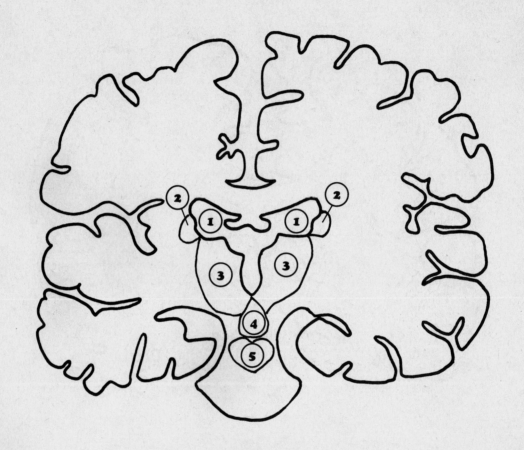

¹Ventricle
²Caudate nucleus
³Trigonum
⁴Midbrain
⁵Pons

Fig. 249 CORONAL SECTION OF
THE BRAIN

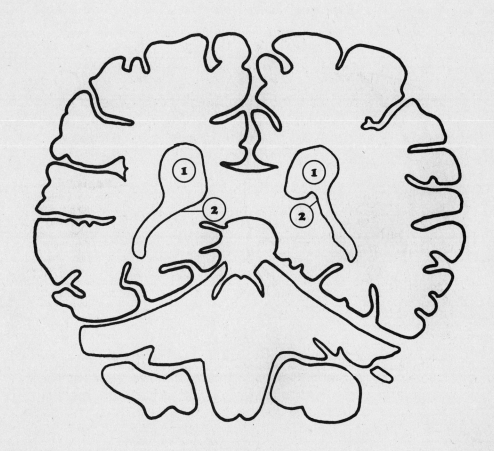

¹Lateral ventricle
²Choroid plexus

Fig. 250 SAGITTAL PLANE THROUGH THE SKULL

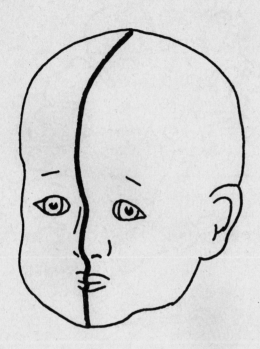

Sagittal Section

The sagittal section is made by rotating the coronal plane 90° (Fig. 250). The midline section demonstrates the corpus callosum and cavum septi pellucidi. The third ventricle lies below the corpus callosum with the massa intermedia. The aqueduct joins the third ventricle to the fourth ventricle (Fig. 251). The section to each side of the midline demonstrates the lateral ventricle, the caudate nuclei, and the choroid plexus (Fig. 252).

Fig. 251 FOURTH VENTRICLE☆

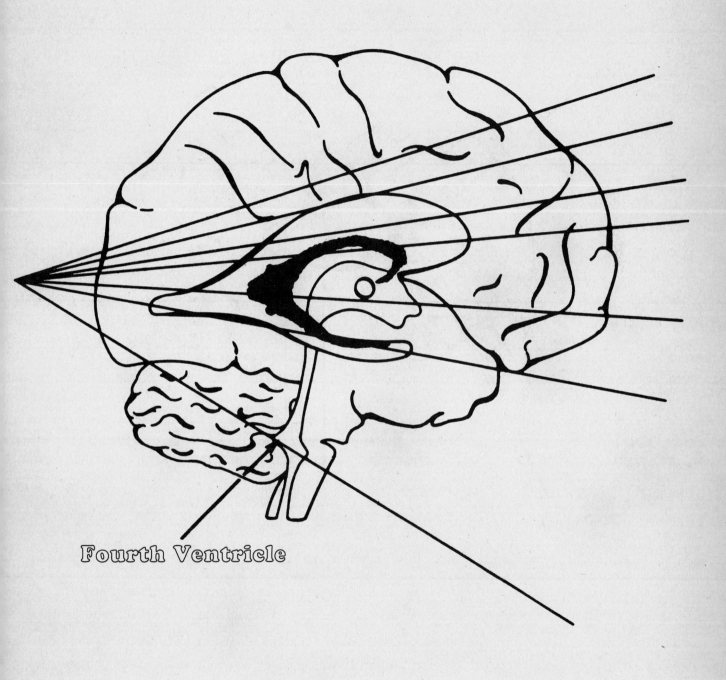

Fourth Ventricle

☆ The pie-shaped lines represent a theoretical ultrasound transducer pathway through the neonatal skull.

Fig. 252 SAGITTAL VIEW OF THE LATERAL VENTRICLE☆

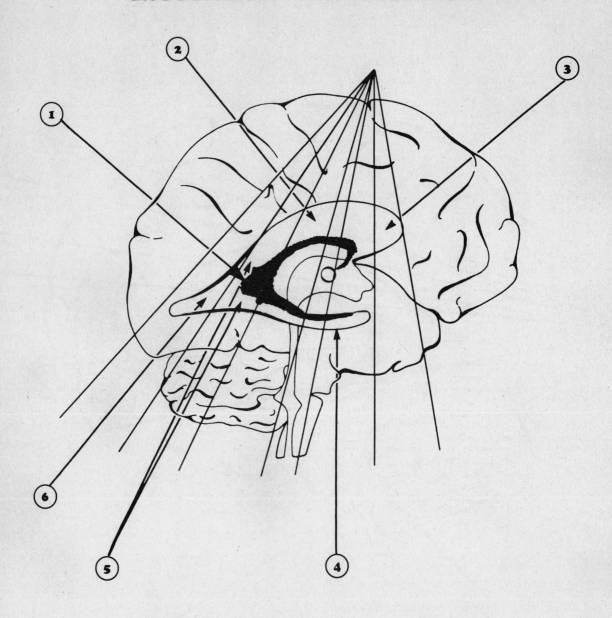

¹Glomus choroideum
²Body of the lateral ventricle
³Anterior horn
⁴Inferior horn
⁵Atrium
⁶Posterior horn

☆ The pie-shaped lines represent a theoretical ultrasound transducer pathway through the neonatal skull.

272

Fig. 253 AXIAL PLANE THROUGH THE SKULL

Axial Section

The brain is sliced from one lateral side to the other parallel to the canthomeatal line (Fig. 253). The first section is made 15° to 20° above the canthomeatal line. The cerebellum is seen posteriorly as it is separated from the cerebrum by the tentorium (Fig. 254). A section 5 mm above the external auditory meatus demonstrates the ambient cisterns between the hippocampal gyrus and the cerebral peduncle and inferior colliculi (Fig. 255). A slice slightly more superior shows the thalami as symmetrical structures on each side of the midline (Fig. 256). The third ventricle lies between the thalami. The frontal horns of the lateral ventricles are anterior to the thalami. The caudate nucleus is found posterolateral to each frontal horn. The occipital horns of the lateral ventricles are posterior to the thalami, and the interhemispheric fissure lies between the occipital horns and frontal horns.

The body of the lateral ventricles can be seen in a section approximately 15 mm to 20 mm above the external auditory meatus (Figs. 257 and 258). The corpus callosum is seen between the lateral ventricles. The caudate nuclei lie in the lateral walls of the ventricles. The choroid plexus is seen within the lateral ventricles.

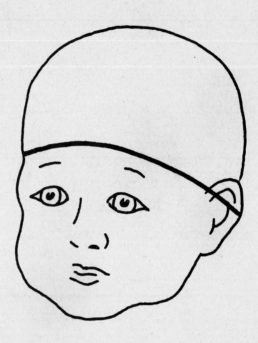

Fig. 254 AXIAL SECTION OF THE BRAIN AT THE LEVEL OF THE EXTERNAL AUDITORY MEATUS

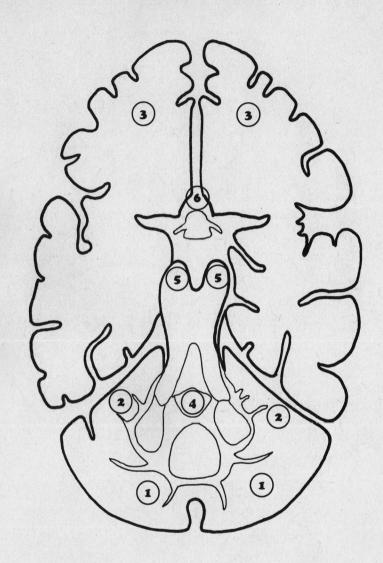

¹Cerebellum
²Tentorium
³Cerebrum
⁴Fourth ventricle
⁵Cerebral peduncle
⁶Circle of Willis

Fig. 255 AXIAL SECTION OF THE BRAIN 5 mm ABOVE THE EXTERNAL AUDITORY MEATUS

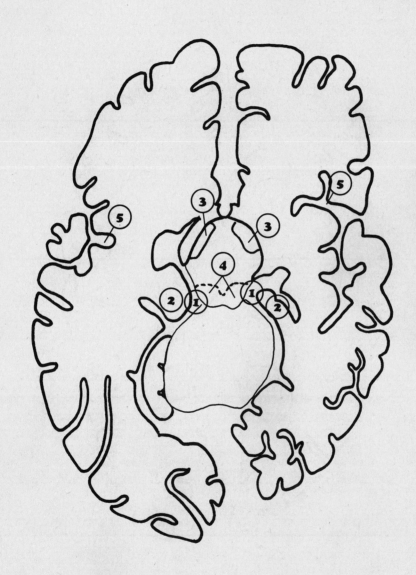

[1] Ambient cistern
[2] Hippocampal gyrus
[3] Cerebral peduncle
[4] Inferior colliculus
[5] Sylvian fissure

Fig. 256 AXIAL SECTION OF THE BRAIN 10 mm ABOVE THE EXTERNAL AUDITORY MEATUS

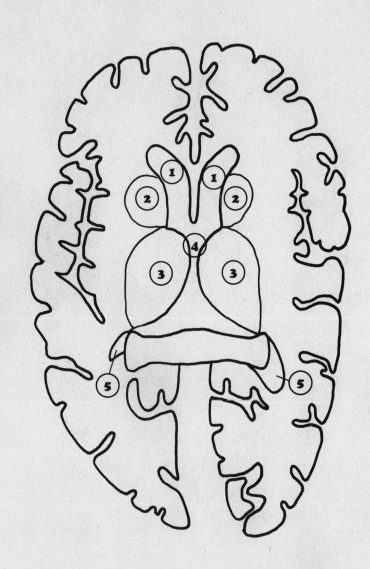

¹Frontal horn
²Caudate nucleus
³Thalamus
⁴Third ventricle
⁵Occipital horn

Fig. 257 AXIAL SECTION OF THE BRAIN 15-20 mm ABOVE THE EXTERNAL AUDITORY MEATUS

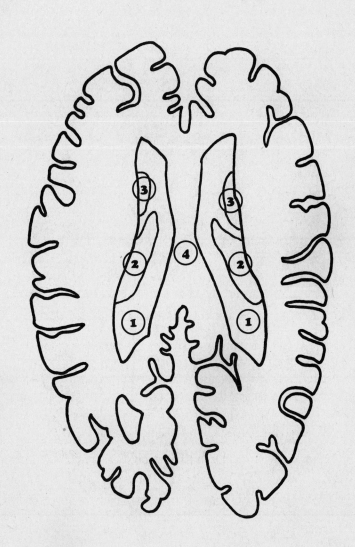

[1]Lateral ventricle
[2]Choroid plexus
[3]Caudate nucleus
[4]Corpus callosum

Fig. 258 AXIAL SECTION OF THE BRAIN 20-25 mm ABOVE THE CANTHOMEATAL LINE

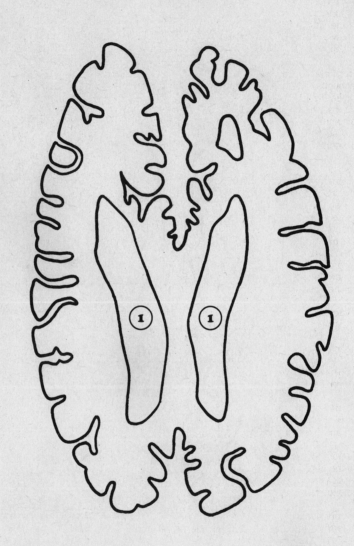

[1]Lateral ventricle

Fig. 259 STRUCTURE OF THE EYE

EYE

Eyeball (Fig. 259)

The eyeball is a spheroid located in the anterior part of the orbit. It consists of anterior and posterior portions and has three layers. The outer layer of the posterior portion is a tough connective tissue layer, the sclera. This is continuous anteriorly with the cornea, which is transparent and covers the portion of the eye that is seen from the anterior as the pupil and iris. The middle, or vascular, layer is the choroid layer and is continuous anteriorly with the ciliary body and then the colored portion of the eye, the iris.

The internal layer is the retina, which contains a pigmented layer. This is continuous anteriorly as a nonvisual layer that lines the inside surface of the ciliary body and iris. The point at which the visual or optic part and the ciliary or nonvisual part join is the ora serrata.

The vitreous body is the jellylike material that occupies 80% of the eyeball.

The lens is a transparent, biconvex, circular structure that lies on the anterior surface of the vitreous body and posterior to the iris and pupil. The lens consists of many concentric layers surrounded by an elastic capsule and is held in position by suspensory ligaments.

The portion of the eye between the transparent cornea anteriorly and the iris posteriorly is the anterior chamber of the eye and contains aqueous humor. The anterior chamber is connected directly with the posterior chamber via the pupillary opening. The posterior chamber of the eye is between the iris anteriorly and the lens and its suspensory ligament posteriorly.

The eyeball is supplied by three sets of ciliary arteries: the short posterior ciliary, the long posterior ciliary, and the anterior ciliary arteries. It is also supplied by a very important artery to the retina.

The large venae vorticosae pierce the sclera just posterior to the equator; they arise from a complex of veins in the choroid layer and empty into the ophthalmic veins.

The central retinal artery usually enters the optic nerve at some point anterior to the optic foramen. It enters the retina at the optic disc and immediately branches into a superior and inferior vessel.

The retinal veins correspond to the arteries and converge on the optic disc to enter the optic nerve.

The nerves to the eyeball are the short and long ciliary nerves and the optic nerve.

Lacrimal Apparatus

The lacrimal apparatus consists of the lacrimal gland and its ducts, the conjunctiva, the lacrimal puncta and canaliculi, and the lacrimal sac and nasolacrimal duct.

The lacrimal gland lies in the lacrimal fossa on the superior lateral aspect of the anterior part of the orbit. It has several ducts that open into the superior fornix of the conjunctiva. Fluid is constantly produced by the lacrimal glands and is spread evenly over the conjunctiva by blinking of the eylids.

Muscles of the Orbit

The voluntary muscles contained in the orbit are the levator palpebrae superioris, the superior rectus, the inferior rectus, the medial rectus, the lateral rectus, the superior oblique, and the inferior oblique.

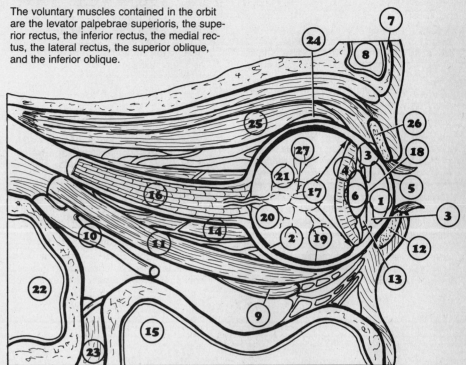

1 Aqueous chamber
2 Choroid
3 Ciliary muscle
4 Ciliary processes
5 Cornea
6 Crystalline lens
7 Frontal bone
8 Frontal sinus
9 Inferior oblique muscle
10 Inferior ophthalmic vein
11 Inferior rectus muscle
12 Inferior tarsus
13 Iris
14 Lateral rectus muscle
15 Maxillary sinus
16 Optic nerve
17 Ora serrata
18 Pupil of the iris
19 Retina
20 Retinal artery and vein
21 Sclera
22 Sphenoid sinus
23 Pterygopalatine ganglion
24 Superior oblique muscle
25 Superior rectus muscle
26 Superior tarsus
27 Vitreous chamber

Neck

Fig. 260 ROOT OF THE NECK ON THE RIGHT SIDE OF THE BODY

The neck is divided into various triangles: the posterior triangle, the anterior triangle, and the submandibular triangle. The muscles of these triangles have already been discussed in the section on the muscular system.

The arteries of the posterior triangle consist of the subclavian artery and the thyrocervical trunk (which branches to form the inferior thyroid artery, the suprascapular artery, and the transversae colli artery) (Fig. 260).

The arteries of the anterior triangle consist of the common carotid artery. This artery is a major branch of the brachiocephalic artery on the right, or the arch of the aorta on the left. The common carotid further divides into the internal and external carotid arteries.

The internal jugular vein emerges from the skull at the jugular foramen, together with the vagus nerve, and close to the internal carotid artery where it enters the carotid canal. Along with the internal and external carotid arteries, the internal jugular vein and vagus nerve de-scend in a fibrous envelope, the carotid sheath, to leave the anterior triangle by passing deep to the sternomastoid muscle.

The submandibular gland is a major salivary gland. It is palpable as a soft mass over the posterior portion of the mylohyoid muscle.

MIDLINE STRUCTURES

The cartilaginous skeleton of the larynx and trachea forms a set of landmarks to which other structures of the midline of the neck can be related:

Hyoid bone: a horseshoe-shaped bone with a central body and greater and lesser horns

Larynx: The skeleton of the larynx consists of a group of cartilaginous structures at the level of cervical vertebrae 3, 4, 5, and 6.

Thyroid cartilage: consists of two flat plates, or laminae, joined anteriorly in the midline. Each lamina has a superior and an inferior cornu and on its lateral surface, a raised oblique line.

Cricoid cartilage: has the shape of a signet ring, with the wide part posteriorly. It provides a posterior point of articulation for the inferior horn or the thyroid cartilage.

Pharynx: a tube that serves both respiratory and digestive functions. It extends inferiorly from posterior to the nose to the level of the cricoid cartilage.

Esophagus: the superior portion of the digestive tube. It commences at the level of the cricoid cartilage and passes posteriorly to the trachea on an inferior course to the thoracic inlet.

Recurrent larynegeal nerve: a branch of the vagus nerve running in the groove between the trachea and esophagus and entering the larynx from below. It supplies all of the muscles of the larnyx except one.

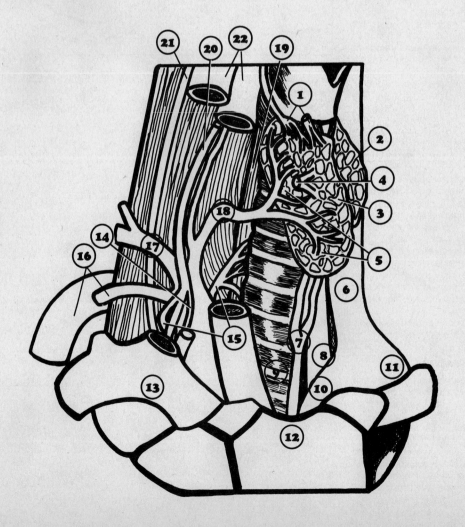

1. Superior thyroid artery and vein
2. Thyroid gland, left lobe
3. Thyroid gland, right lobe pulled anteriorly
4. Middle thyroid vein
5. Parathyroid glands
6. Left internal jugular vein
7. Inferior thyroid veins
8. Left common carotid artery
9. Trachea
10. Left brachiocephalic vein
11. Subclavian vein
12. Suprasternal notch
13. Subclavian, vertebral, and right brachiocephalic veins
14. Cardiac branch of the vagus nerve
15. Recurrent laryngeal nerve
16. Subclavian and suprascapular arteries
17. Transverse cervical artery
18. Inferior thyroid artery
19. Esophagus
20. Vagus nerve and ascending cervical artery
21. Phrenic nerve on the anterior scalene muscle
22. Internal jugular vein and common carotid artery

Fig. 261 CROSS SECTION OF THE NECK AT THE LEVEL OF THE 5th CERVICAL VERTEBRA

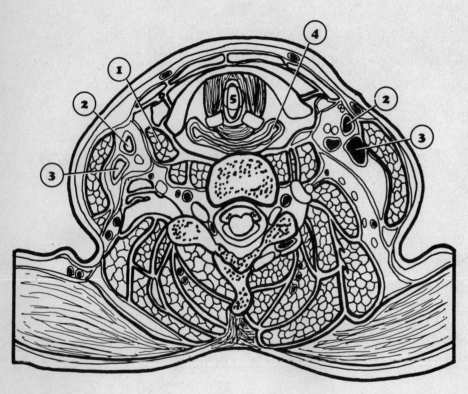

THYROID GLAND

The thyroid gland consists of a right and left lobe connected in the midline by an isthmus. Each lobe is bounded posterolaterally by the carotid artery and internal jugular vein and is lateral to the trachea (Figs. 261 and 262). The sternocleidomastoid and strap muscles (sternothyroid, sternohyoid, and omohyoid) are situated anterolateral to the thyroid gland.

The right lobe is often the larger of the two lobes. The isthmus lies anterior to the trachea and may be variable in size. A triangular cephalic extension of the isthmus, the pyramidal lobe, is present in 15% to 30% of thyroid glands. When present, it is of varying size and is more commonly found on the left. A fibrous capsule encloses the gland and gives it a smooth contour.

Blood is supplied to the thyroid via four arteries. Two superior thyroid arteries arise from the external carotids and descend to the upper poles. Two inferior thyroid arteries arise from the thyrocervical trunk of the subclavian artery and ascend to the lower poles. The corresponding veins drain into the internal jugular vein.

Parathyroid Glands

The parathyroid glands are four small endocrine glands that secrete a hormone important in the metabolism of calcium. They are embedded in the posterior wall of the capsule of the thyroid gland.

¹Thyroid
²Carotid artery
³Jugular vein
⁴Pharynx
⁵Rima glottidis

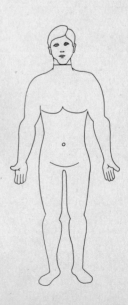

Fig. 262 CROSS SECTION OF THE NECK AT THE LEVEL OF THE 7th CERVICAL VERTEBRA

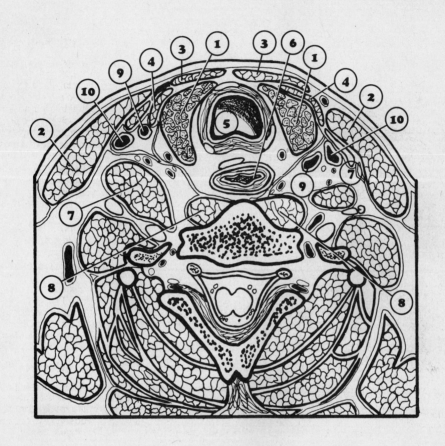

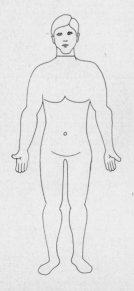

¹Thyroid
²Sternocleidomastoid muscle
³Sternohyoid muscle
⁴Sternothyroid muscle
⁵Trachea
⁶Esophagus
⁷Scalenus anterior muscle
⁸Longus colli muscle
⁹Carotid artery
¹⁰Jugular vein

BIBLIOGRAPHY

Anderson PD: Clinical Anatomy and Physiology for Allied Health Sciences. Philadelphia, WB Saunders, 1976

Bejar R, Coen R: Normal cranial ultrasonography in neonates. In James HE, Anas NG, Perkin RM (eds): Brain Insults in Infants and Children: Pathophysiology and Management. Orlando, Grune & Stratton, 1985

Crafts RC: A Textbook of Human Anatomy, 2nd ed. New York, John Wiley & Sons, 1979

Hagen-Ansert, SL: Textbook of Diagnostic Ultrasonography, 2nd ed. Chapters: High-resolution ultrasonography of superficial structures (Schorzman L); Breast (Ezo L, Hagen-Ansert SL); Ultrasound evaluation of the neonatal skull (Appareti K et al). St. Louis, CV Mosby, 1983

Hollinshead WH: Textbook of Anatomy, 3rd ed. Philadelphia, Harper & Row, 1982

Introduction to Medical Sciences for Clinical Practice, Unit XIII: Obstetrics. Chicago, Year Book Medical Publishers, 1977

Kapit W, Elson LM: The Anatomy Coloring Book. New York, Harper & Row, 1977

Lyons, EA: A Color Atlas of Sectional Anatomy. St. Louis, C. V. Mosby, 1978

Moore, KL: The Developing Human. Philadelphia, WB Saunders, 1973

Netter FH: The CIBA Collection of Medical Illustrations, Vol. 3: Digestive system, Part III: Liver, biliary tract and pancreas. Summit, NJ, CIBA, 1977

Netter FH: The CIBA Collection of Medical Illustrations, Vol. 5: Heart. Summit, NJ, CIBA, 1974

Pernkopf E: Atlas of Topographical and Applied Human Anatomy, Vol. 2. Philadelphia, WB Saunders, 1964

Rumack CM, Johnson ML: Perinatal and Infant Brain Imaging. Chicago, Year Book Medical Publishers, 1984

Sahn DJ, Anderson F: Two-Dimensional Anatomy of the Heart. New York, John Wiley & Sons, 1982

Snell RS: Clinical Anatomy for Medical Students. Boston, Little, Brown & Co, 1973

Thompson JS: Core Textbook of Anatomy. Philadelphia, JB Lippincott, 1977